Power to
the Patient

For information about special discounts for bulk purchases, please contact:
info@VesaliusPress.com or
Barbara@TheMedicalStrategist.com

ISBN-10: 0615511821
EAN-13: 9780615511825

Power to the Patient

Barbara Hales, M.D.

Dedications and Acknowledgement

This book is dedicated to my colleagues in all specialties and to my patients who have shown me how to truly care for others while becoming a better physician...and a better person. We are currently at a crossroads of healthcare and as we adapt to the changing landscape of medicine, we are all learning as we move forward.

A special dedication goes to my precious family—Jonathan Stuart, Justine Alyssa and David Brandon who have given me the true meaning of life and how to live it.

Copyright and Legal Notice

© 2011 Barbara Hales, M.D.

All rights reserved

Published under the Copyright Laws of the Library of Congress of The U.S.A. by:

Vesalius Press
Boynton Beach, Florida

info@VesaliusPress.com

www.VesaliusPress.com

Foreword

Thank you Dr. Hales for the new masterpiece, *"Power to the Patient"*. After eight years as a partner in a prestigious Wall Street "think tank", I have spent the last 24 years as an executive and leader on the business side of healthcare. Physicians, groups, hospitals, IPAs and payers depend on my advice in making forward thinking strategic business decisions. I don't say this to impress you, but rather to impress upon you how overwhelmed I am with the work on this project.

Never has there been a timelier, more in depth report that fairly provides all angles, as viewed from all participants, in the nation's most misunderstood industry. Though your target market by the title appears to be the patient, I believe this should be required reading for everyone involved in providing healthcare, no matter what their level or profession within the office or hospital. I found your presentation and balance of clarifying complicated concepts and systems to be just remarkable.

Congratulations on this fantastic, "must read" primer. From patient to back office worker, clarification and understanding is now at your fingertips. Count on me to tell everyone I know and work with about this landmark effort. Never has there been such a disconnect as that which exists between the patient and the healthcare provider. Thank you for bridging that gap.

Doug Sparks - Co-Founder MD/PT Partners
www.mdptpartners.com

Contents

Integrative Medicine, Evidence-Based Medicine, The Mind-Body Connection

Current Status of US Health Care, Preventable Deaths: Lifestyle Choices, Emerging Models of Health Care, Power to the People

Introduction:
Patient Empowerment

Patient Empowerment, Healing Traditions,
Healthcare versus Sickcare,
The Internet and Health, Trends

Patient empowerment, personalized medicine, integrative medicine...health care is undergoing a radical transformation. Dr. Andrew Weil says that the health care system as we know it is in total economic collapse, that medical institutions are imploding, and that market forces and consumer demand are dragging conventional medicine, kicking and screaming, into a new perspective of health care. [1]

Every social institution operates on a natural cycle of ebb and flow. Scientific thought swells outward, embraces new ideas, and then recedes, narrowing its focus to study the particulars and then again, spills out to influence the wider perspective.

Institutions, by their nature, are resistant to change and the changes occurring in medicine and health care are the focus of many criticisms. The growing acceptance of complementary and alternative therapies, the use of the Internet for health information, the move from a pharmaceutically-driven health market to a model based on truly preventive medicine...the long specialized and stagnant health care system is getting an injection of holistic thinking and a shaking up of the balances of power.

Conventional medicine, as it is perceived today, is based on "evidence-based research," symptoms and the drugs to treat them, technology and specialization. But medicine hasn't always been so fragmented or so narrow.

Historically, medicine has included a wider perspective: healing based on interconnectedness, healing that includes diet, lifestyle and cleansing, health as it relates to a whole person's life, morality and spirituality, community and balances of nature.

Today, more people and more doctors are coming to understand that health care isn't about treating a symptom but about treating a disease. It's not about taking a drug but about identifying and changing the factors that contribute to medical conditions. It's not about treating just a condition but about treating a whole person, and the personal and cultural factors that play a part in health.

At the root of these changes is the growing trend for people to take their health into their own hands. They're distrustful of a pharmaceutically-driven system; they're distrustful of government positions and recommendations that have proven false; they're not waiting to be told what's right for them anymore: they're finding out for themselves.

Eight in ten of the Americans using the Internet have used it to look up health information, according to the 2005 Pew findings, with the focus increasingly shifting from searching for symptoms and specific conditions to growing interest in diet, fitness, experimental treatments, particular doctors and hospitals and drug and health insurance information. [2]

Thomas Goetz, executive editor of *Wired Magazine* and author of **Decision Tree**, describes the early research concerning health and empowerment conducted in 1967. [3] Michael Marmot and Geoffrey Rise looked at the rates of heart disease in 18,000 civil servants in a London School of Hygiene and Tropical Medicine and University College study. [3] The researchers found that social rank was the greatest indicator of death due to heart disease: those lowest on the totem pole were *four times* as likely to die from the disease than their work superiors. [3]

When they investigated further, and qualified the results, accounting for unhealthy habits like smoking, exercise and unhealthy eating; they were surprised to learn that 60% of the deaths could not be attributed to these factors.

Instead, Marmot proposed that control, the degree of power and/or helplessness each participant encountered, was the dividing difference between the subjects. The workers that had lower social status also had less control over their own lives and destinies, said Marmot in his book **The Status Syndrome**, and it was this fact more than any other, that affected people's health. [3]

Goetz writes about the personalized medicine trend taking place today: Internet-use and consumer technologies that are freeing people from paternalistic medicine, the research in genetics, molecular science and bioinformatics that are putting preventive medicine and medical knowledge in the hands of many, and the increasing realization that knowledge is power—in more ways than one.

Chapter 1:
Preventive Medicine As It's Been

*Band-Aids and Magic Bullets, Fear-Mongering
and Pharmaceutical Companies,
The Creation of Illness, Iatrogenics*

Conventional medicine today is full of blanket warnings and magic bullets, pills for every symptom and a name for every possible condition. CAT scans, blood tests, genotyping... there's a test for everything and a prediction around every corner.

Yet with all the advances in medicine and health technology, we get less personalized care than any time in medical history and our faith in science has been exploited by the pharmaceutical industry to sell us more medications than ever.

Medicalization, disease-mongering, fear-mongering, the worried well...these are more terms that are common in today's health industry. The greed behind many of the health messages that we get is starting to backfire. When a culture is long-consumed with health fears; it only makes sense that it begins to question the sources of those health conditions, the treatments that have or haven't helped and the credibility of the messengers.

A Culture of Convenience

One of the reasons the health care industry, as a "sick care" industry, has become so entrenched is because of cultural ideas about science. Science, for most of us, is something we think of as making our lives easier: processed foods that cut short our time in the kitchen, prescriptions that stand in for lengthy medical evaluations and every form of shopping available from home and at our fingertips.

We're a consumer culture and we've been market-branded since birth to keep it that way. We get our ideas about what is valuable, what status entails, what health and happiness are— from the world of media.

And we want "the magic bullet," the pill that will clear everything up, the bottled wonder that will make all of our unhealthy lifestyle practices moot.

Thomas Goetz says that lurking behind the idea of personalized medicine are the futuristic dreams, heightened by television programs, about instant scans and perfect diagnoses that science will bring us: a Star Trek or Jetson's kind of technology. [4]

Fulfilling those expectations, so far, has come in the way of drugs, says Goetz. But the problem is, drugs aren't personal, they're not specific to individuals, they're meant to serve as many people as generally as possible.

This is why compounding pharmacies have come under fire for mixing bio-identical hormone treatments that are tailored specifically to the needs of an individual: you can't patent natural substances, you can't patent a medication made for one and you're certainly not going to make money off of it even if you could.

That doesn't mean it won't be attempted: in 2001, Big Pharma was fined $871 million for conspiring to jack up the price of natural substances, vitamins. [10]

Drug dependence is why more health conditions are emerging every day, why more drugs are created to treat this symptom or that, why the pharmaceutical industry, with their influence over doctors, insurance companies, the media and government agencies, is creating a culture of the "worried well."

A "sick-care" system is a profitable one. Preventive medicine, personalized medicine, medical homes and doctor teams: these are all big threats to profiteers in health care.

The Worried Well

The pharmaceutical industry has always spent a lot of money on sponsoring research that suits them, creating health information news stories that they sell to TV news stations, magazines and newspapers, paying for the bulk of advertisements in medical journals and both directly and indirectly targeting doctors and medical journalists with sales representatives, continuing education programs and sponsorship programs but nowadays: they're going straight for the consumer.

Alison Bass, author of **Side Effects: A Prosecuter, a Whistleblower and a Bestselling Antidepressant on Trial**, says that there are so many drug advertisements on American TV today for one simple fact: they work. [6]

Duke University's Ruth Day and her colleagues studied drug advertisements and found that producers use a number of tactics to detract from possible side effects and compromise the whole message. [6]

A Nasonex commercial uses an animated, flying and flashing bee, for instance, to distract the viewer's attention when possible side effects are mentioned, a bee that hovers respectfully to the side when the potential benefits are listed. [6]

Marketing budgets have bloomed in terms of directly targeting consumers, twice as fast as that which is spent on doctors and research shows that they increase patient's request for the drugs and the likelihood that their doctor will give them out. [5]

Iona Heath, a general practitioner published an article titled "Who Needs Health Care—The Well or the Sick?" in a 2005 issue of the *British Medical Journal (BMJ)*. Heath points out that the more money, the more education, and the more health a society has; the higher the rates of self-reported illness. [9] American citizens, with higher rates of exposure to doctors and modern health care, report feeling sicker than the poorest state in India with the highest death rates. [9]

Heath says that three trends: the industrialization of health, the medicalization of life and the politicization of medicine combine to give a unique version of preventive medicine, one that causes healthy people to worry about *keeping* well, one that stresses unnecessary and expensive screenings and drug-taking that increases the risk of medically-caused illness and death. [9]

These are the worried well.

Fear-mongering makes healthy people "medical consumers." It expands the market and "medicalizing" normal life conditions extends the life of a drug patent. [5]

If a drug can be used to treat new symptoms; manufacturers get another long-term lock on profits. [5] Paxil was rejuvenated in this way to treat social anxiety disorder. The product director of the drug was quoted as saying: "Every marketer's dream is to find an unidentified or unknown market and develop it. That's what we were able to do with Social Anxiety Disorder." [5]

Indeed, the pharmaceutical industry spends more on marketing than on research and development. Creating "disease awareness" and "medicalizing" life is a way to widen the market. [7]

Medicalization is a term coined in the 1970's: it entails turning common ailments into conditions requiring treatment, defining risks as actual diseases and skewing prevalence and statistics to make the new condition sound more imminent and more dangerous than it actually is. [7]

Philosopher Ivan Illich criticized our medical system for claiming "authority over people who are not yet ill, people who cannot reasonably expect to get well, and those for whom doctors have no more effective treatment than that which could be offered by their uncles or aunts." [8]

Disease-mongering was described in the 1990's by medical writer Lynn Payer as the double-exploitation of citizen's anxieties about health and their faith in science in order to re-cruit a wider drug market. [7]

Over three decades ago, then-CEO of Merck Pharmaceuticals Henry Gadsen predicted the coming market population in an interview with *Fortune Magazine*. He wanted drug company products to become as common as chewing gum, to make drugs that would "sell to every-one, sick or healthy." [8]

Vince Parry, global marketing expert and au-thor of "The Art of Branding A Condition," il-lustrates just how accurate Gadsen's prediction was. [8] Parry specializes in helping Big Pharma create new diseases. [8]

Parry outlines how to do this: give an old disease a new name or expand its definition; revive a little-known (and rarely experienced) condition and make it sound widespread and imminent; create a whole new condition from risk factors. [8]

Osteoporosis is a symptom of aging that we now think of as a disease; high cholesterol level is a risk factor that is now considered a condition that needs treatment; bad breath or "halitosis" was first medicalized by Listerine commercials. [8]

Alan Cassels and Ray Moynihan report on many of these issues in their *Le Monde diplomatique* article: "US: Selling to the Worried Well. [6]

The writers describe a *Reuters Business Insights* report in which drug company executives were challenged to convince the public that "problems they may previously have accepted as, perhaps, merely an inconvenience" are actually medical conditions that require treatment. [8]

The *Reuters* report, talking about surging profits, said: "The coming years will bear great witness to the corporate-sponsored creation of disease." [8]

While the marketers expand definitions of disease, they simultaneously splinter and compress causes to blur the big picture, says Cassels and Moynihan. [8] Forget the real causes of heart disease (processed foods, stress, smoking, physical inactivity etc.) and worry about cholesterol levels, take drugs to lower (or keep) your blood pressure low. Your unhappiness doesn't have to do with your stress levels or life choices: it's an imbalance of neurotransmitters in your brain. [8]

Yet our pill-popping tendencies have a cost.

Ivan Illich said that our medical system undermines "the human capacity to cope with the reality of suffering and death." [8]

True, generations of people are growing up with one "happy pill" or another, used to eradicate uncomfortable emotions or make children docile—we can easily become "comfortably numb."

Antibiotic over-use, by both consumers and industrial producers of animal products, has created superbugs.

And the worst of it? The Nutrition Institute of America recently did a quality review of "government-approved" medicine and found that iatrogenesis, death caused by conventional medical treatment, is actually *the leading cause of mortality in the U.S.* [10]

Iatrogenic Deaths

In 2006, professors Gary Null and Dorothy Smith, along with doctors Carolyn Dean, Martin Feldman and Debora Rasio published the results of their review and titled it: "Death By Medicine." [10]

What did they find?

- 2.2 million people have adverse reactions to prescription drugs, requiring hospitalization, every year in America

- 20 million antibiotic prescriptions are given for viral infections (with which they have no effect) every year

- 7.5 million unnecessary medical and surgical procedures are performed annually

- 8.9 million people are unnecessarily hospitalized every year

- 800, 000 Americans die due to modern medical practice every year

The authors also estimated the deaths that would occur over a 10-year span and found:

- 1.06 million Americans will die from an adverse drug reaction

- 0.98 million will die of medical errors

- 1.15 million people will die of bedsores

- 0.88 million people will die from infections caused by hospital or medical treatments

- 1.09 million people will die of malnutrition caused by medical treatments or lack of nursing staff

- 1.99 of us will die due to outpatient treatments

- 371, 360 Americans will die because of unnecessary procedures

- 320,000 deaths will occur due to surgery

Their prediction of more than 7.8 million iatrogenic deaths in just 10 years is, the authors say, a number more than all the casualties of all the wars the US has ever engaged in, combined. [10]

The researchers also point out that the numbers are likely much higher: "as few as 5% and no more than 20% of iatrogenic events are ever reported." [10]

Health versus Wealth

The most damning evidence that our health care system is about profit and not people comes from trade agreements and drug patent protection.

Huge numbers of people in developing countries die every day of illnesses that American drug companies could easily combat but saving lives is just not as profitable as selling unnecessary drugs to healthy Americans. Worse yet, the industry claims intellectual rights to research and formulations to prevent other scientists from developing generic versions of these drugs to save lives in poorer nations.

The French newspaper *Le Monde diplomatique* calls this "apartheid of pharmacology." [5] *The Guardian* says that much more profit is gleaned from treating "diseases of affluence and longevity" than battling true disease and mortality. [5]

In 1995, the drug giant Aventis discontinued production of the only safe medication for the fatal stage of sleeping sickness because it wasn't a profitable market. [5] Then, in 2000, the drug was used as a money-generating hair-removing cream in the West. [5] Only after much public outcry and legal wrangling did Aventis donate the drug to the World Health Organization and agree to help fund research and treatment programs. [5]

The pharmaceutical industry is growing at three times the rate of Fortune 500 companies and the fact that the U.S. is the only First World nation that doesn't control drug prices certainly helps in this regard. [5]

The global pharmaceutical market is expected to bring in over a trillion dollars by 2012. [11]

The U.S. drug industry owned 42.8% of this revenue in 2007 with profits of $315 billion. [11, 12]

The industry spent $6.3 million in just the latter half of the last quarter to lobby Congress, the White House and federal agencies during health care reform. [13] In 2007, the industry spent a total of $168 million on lobbying. [14] In 1998, the drug industry in America spent $12 million on campaign contributions. [5]

The revenue it accrues, says the industry, is used to pay for research and development and is why patent rights are so crucial. [5] But, as Noam Chomsky, author of **Unsustainable Development** says, most research is paid for by the public—almost half—and the basic biology and science is also publicly funded. [5]

Wayne M. O'Leary, author of **The Real Drug Lords**, says that data compiled by the National Bureau of Economic Research reported that 15 of the 21 most beneficial drugs were introduced due to public—not private—research between 1965 and 1992. [5]

He adds that estimates through the 1990's put drug discovery research by the drug industry at the range of 17 to 40%, the remainder were performed by National Institutes of Health researchers, nonprofits and universities. [5]

AIDS activist Jamie Love questions the right of Big Pharma to own drug rights to begin with. [5] Many pricey AIDS treatments were developed out of existing government research on cancer—research the public has already invested in. He asks: How is it that drug companies are awarded the moral authority to decide who gets drugs and who doesn't? [5]

When Jonas Salk, inventor of the polio vaccine, was asked why he never sought a patent; he answered "Could you patent the sun?" [5]

Vermont Senator Patrick Leahy introduced "The Public Research in the Public Interest Act" in 2006. [15] Billions of tax dollars go to universities to "outsource" medical research every year. [15] Although these are public funds, the schools then hold exclusive patent rights that they often license to private industries, a practice that can worsen monopolization of drugs and technology. [15]

Leahy proposed that all federally-funded research patents be open to generic competition in developing countries, a market that wouldn't affect the U.S. drug market. [15] This was too slippery a slope however, even for life-saving medicines, and the act didn't pass. [15]

As J.W.Smith, author of **The World's Wasted Wealth 2,** wrote: "There is a direct conflict between the pursuit of health and the pursuit of wealth."

Chapter 2: Trust in Medicine

*Trust in Government Recommendations,
Trust in Government Regulation*

Trust is the real issue at stake today. Trust is social capital: it's the glue that holds a society together and it's the real source of healing in any medical relationship. When we believe that our doctor cares for us, when we believe that our government is actively guarding our well-being, when our expectation is that we will get better: we often do.

That's not just any hokey principle: it's the basis of mind-body medicine; it's the basis of the placebo effect.

Research has shown that faith isn't always a conscious thing: we all hold subconscious associations about doctors, medicine and pain. A doctor's white coat, a stethoscope, the disinfectant smell of an examining room: all of these things trigger conditioned responses that are emotional, mental and physiological. [29]

What we think, what we feel and what we experience physically aren't distinct from one another: think tension headaches or indigestion caused by stress; consider what thoughts are running in the back of your mind the next time you feel frustrated or sad.

Advancing technology gives basis to the placebo effect and evidence that mind-body medicine works. It's why cognitive behavioral therapy (CBT) is useful for depression, why functional Magnetic Resonance Imaging (fMRI) is effective for managing pain. Accessing our thoughts and making use of them affects immune responses and hormone function. [29] We can learn to control activity in certain regions of the brain.

A recent survey conducted by the National Institutes of Health (NIH) found that 46 to 58% of doctors admit to regularly using placebos. [27] That might seem shocking, but confidence and faith are the foundation of medicine. It's the respect and trust that we've learned to associate with the profession that makes us more likely to heal.

"The placebo effect can be engendered without any pill at all by the positivity and the personality of the physician...by simply talking to patients and reassuring them and empathizing with them," says Dr. W. Grant Thompson, author of **The Placebo Effect and Health**. [28]

"The mere handing of a pill to a patient is a shortcut for this and often, I believe, would not be necessary if physicians took time to communicate with patients about their experience of illness." [28]

Today, our health care system has compromised our faith in our doctors. They've been made the middle men, forced to see as many patients as they can and forced to fill quotas for treatments and profit. They're torn between the scientific foundation of their profession and the emerging evidence that holistic medicine is where it's at. They're compromised by the drug industry and managed care systems and are forced to treat patients like commodities rather than people.

And government? The Pew Research Center has just published results of a poll that finds faith in the US government at an all-time low. [31] 8 in 10 Americans don't trust the government and don't expect that it can solve our problems. [31] Half of the polled citizens said that government "negatively affects their daily lives." [31]

Pew director Andrew Kohut said "Politics has poisoned the well." [31]

The whole "business" of medicine has eroded trust. Blanket recommendations, one-size-fits-all thinking...it's Americans demanding easy cures and general advisories and our carefully-cultured beliefs that a pill will solve all our ills that contribute to the failure of health care today.

But blanket recommendations don't work and no one can predict how this medication or that treatment will work for many when illness is a highly individual and highly complex phenomenon.

Our trust that the government guards our well-being and our faith in the magic pill have been eroded by the "transparency" or increasing amounts of information that are now available to us.

Trust in Government Recommendations

Many people still believe the health recommendations they see or hear in the media, even though these are often sponsored or even created by the pharmaceutical industry.

Scientists and government agencies aren't immune to market pressures either, and their recommendations often become entrenched in the minds of Americans even though scant evidence supports the advisories.

Take the long-standing position the government has taken on fat in the diet.

Fat

Saturated fats were demonized in America for decades as the processed food industry was taking off and polyunsaturated oils, margarines and other substitutes came into being. [17] As the U.S. government told its citizens that saturated fats and animal fats were at the root of high rates of heart disease, as consumption of these fats fell and dietary intake of processed vegetable oils rose, so did the rates of heart disease *rise*. [17]

Early results of the famous Framingham Heart Study were often used as evidence of the connection between fats and heart disease. Forty years later, however, the study director admitted: "In Framingham, Mass, the more saturated fat one ate, the more cholesterol one ate, the more calories one ate, the lower the person's serum cholesterol...we found that the people who ate the most cholesterol, ate the most saturated fat, ate the most calories, weighed the least and were the most physically active." [17]

The American Cancer Society, the National Cancer Institute and the Senate Committee on Nutrition and Human Needs have all held the position that animal fats are linked with both heart disease and cancer but when University of Maryland researchers reviewed the data that was used to support these positions, they found that vegetable fat consumption was linked to increased rates of cancer—and saturated fats were not. [17]

Cholesterol, long touted as a risk factor for heart disease and treated like an actual disease itself, has mysterious links to heart disease—and not clear-cut ones.

Oxidized cholesterol, such as that which is found in processed products subject to high heat, can trigger heart disease but normal cholesterol acts as an antioxidant in the body and is necessary for a whole host of cell, tissue, hormone and neurotransmitter production and many bodily functions. [17]

Lately, "the French Paradox" and the Mediterranean Diet are the basis for new recommendations after decades of study have found no evidence for the link between fat in the diet and increased rates of heart disease, diabetes and obesity. These traditional diets contain as much as 70% saturated fat.

Doctor George Mann, former Co-Director of the Framingham Study said:

"The diet-heart hypothesis has been repeatedly shown to be wrong, and yet, for complicated reasons of pride, profit and prejudice, the hypothesis continues to be exploited by scientists, fund-raising enterprises, food companies and even governmental agencies. The public is being deceived by the greatest health scam of the century." [17]

Statin Drugs

The cholesterol-lowering drugs statins "are the best-selling medicines in history, used by more than 13 million Americans and an additional 12 million patients around the world, producing $27. 8 billion in sales in 2006," according to a January 2008 issue of *Business Week*. [19]

Official government guidelines advised that 40 million Americans should be taking the drug and some scientists have even suggested that they be put in the water supply. [19]

The pharmaceutical industry has promoted statins for use in a host of other conditions, from Alzheimer's disease and cancer to osteoporosis and arthritis. [20] They've worked on gaining the right to make statins an over-the-counter medication. [20]

So how is it, Lew Rockwell columnist Bill Sardi asks, that recent reviews of the drugs Zetia and Vytorin reveal no health benefits? [19] Even though the statins lowered cholesterol levels, this did not reduce arterial plaque or lower the risk of death. [19]

Dr. James M. Wright published a review in the 2007 edition of *Lancet* in which he could find no evidence for reduced risk of death from heart disease with *any* of the statin drugs. [19]

Sardi charges public health agencies and medical journalists with complicity in the deceptive promotion of statin drugs. [19]

He says that the misleading claim, "statin drugs reduce the risk for a sudden death heart attack by 19%", wouldn't pass Federal Trade Commission guidelines because the "hard numbers "only show an 0.8% reduction. [19] Instead, FDA-administered websites and the National Institutes of Health websites make the claim for the drug industry. [19]

16 million Americans were taking Lipitor in 2004, even though a 1999 study found that 36% of the patients on a high dose experienced side effects and 10% did so on the lowest dose. [20]

Complaints about muscle pain and weakness (the heart is a muscle!) and problems with cognition (such as memory loss) have long been reported with the use of statin drugs but pharmaceutical companies, and plenty of other powers-that-be, claimed that the benefits out-weighed the risks. [19] Instead, it appears, the risks outweigh the benefits almost 2 to 1. [19]

A 2004 study enumerating the benefits of cholesterol-lowering drugs was published in the *New England Journal of Medicine (NEJM).* [19] In the NEJM approved-and-reviewed study, statins were said to lower the risk of a cardiovascular event, even as the publicized data and tables showed otherwise. The NEJM did not add a correction until two years later and has never pulled the article from publication. [19]

Multiple studies have shown that statins either have no effect or *actually raise* the risk of death by heart attack including the 2001 Honolulu Heart Program and the 2002 Prosper study. [20]

Mammograms

All types of screenings have become a favored "preventive medicine" technique among Americans, endorsed by government agencies and disease organizations these procedures a useful way to keep health care costs high. Doctors especially, are often pressured into ordering expensive tests for fear of malpractice suits.

For over twelve years, medical experts have been advising that women under 40 reduce their mammogram screenings but it wasn't until 2009 that an independent panel, the US Preventive Services Task Force, has created a new controversy with similar recommendations. [21]

Studies have found that women with certain DNA mutations are more susceptible to a radiation-caused cancer growth.

In a recent study published in the *Journal of Clinical Oncology*, Dr. David Goldgar has found that radiation may reduce the ability of women with the mutations to repair cell damage that normally occurs with the X-rays. This inability to correct the DNA damage leaves them vulnerable to cancer proliferation. [23]

Another study, presented at the Radiological Society of North America, has found that repeated exposure to low-dose radiation can be dangerous for both at-risk women and younger women. [22]

The meta-analysis, led by Dr. Jansen-van der Weide, found that the benefits of breast cancer screenings may be offset by the risks. [22] The researchers found that mammograms increased the risk of breast cancer in at-risk women by 1.5 times and high-risk women who had five or more mammograms were 2 and ½ times more likely to develop breast cancer. [22]

Inherited DNA defects, however, are at fault for only 5 to 10% of breast cancer cases, so the risks of the average woman are somewhat mysterious. [24] Most DNA damage, says doctors Edward White and Melissa Conrad Stöppler, develop during adulthood from exposure to environmental toxins and other sources of radiation. [24]

Nuclear physicist John Gofman believes that medical radiation is behind 83% of breast cancer cases. [25] A *Lancet* journal publication claims that since mammogram screenings have become common; ductal carcinoma in situ breast cancer cases have increased by 328% in women under the age of 40. [25]

Dr. Russell Blaylock estimates that annual mammograms increase the risk of developing breast cancer by 2%, a risk that increases with subsequent exposures to 10% in five years and 20% in ten. [25]

The Breast Cancer Organization, the National Cancer Institute and the American Cancer Institute still endorse mammogram screenings.

Trust in Regulation

One of the worst betrayals Americans encounter has to do with how intricately tangled politics, federal agencies and health care profiteers are in the U.S.

In many other countries, health is considered a right, not a privilege. Citizen health is not a commodity to be exploited so much as a "social good" that promotes the bonds between members of a healthy (in more ways than medically-termed) society in the same way that degree of trust does.

Before the "Death by Medicine" researchers came up with their results about iatrogenesis, statistics were scattered and buried.

Quality Review

In 1978 by the U.S. Office of Technology Assessment (OTA) reported that: "Only 10 to 20% of all procedures currently used in medical practice have been shown to be efficacious by controlled trial." [10]

In 1995 the OTA compared health system effectiveness of the US and seven other industrialized countries and rated the US low in terms of infant mortality [a common signifier of a lack of preventive medicine], life expectancy and quality of care but high in terms of cost. [10]

In the OTA's final review of the US medical system, they wrote: "There are no mechanisms in place to limit dissemination of technologies, regardless of their clinical value." [10]

The OTA was then disbanded by Congress. [10]

Prescription Drug Prices

When Senator Leahy advocated the traveling to Canada by American citizens to buy prescription drugs at a fraction of U.S. costs; a fictional book emerged about terrorist activity and Canadian pills containing poison. [5]

VP of the drug coalition PhRMA (Pharmaceutical Research and Manufacturers of America) and a political consultant for the lobbying group were involved in the sponsorship of the book. [10]

PhRMA isn't stopping there. In 2003, a pharmaceutical spokesperson confirmed a Canadian news report that the group would be adding $1 million to their lobbying budget to try and "change the Canadian health-care system and eliminate subsidized prescription drug prices enjoyed by Canadians." [16]

As American states try to control drug prices in their individual states, PhRMA launches initiatives to limit reforms.

When California proposed a ballot that would punish companies that refused to discount drugs for the poor; PhRMA worked to defeat the ballot before it even got off the ground. [16] PhRMA VP said, "It's a very bad precedent [for] the leader in the country [to take]. We took it as "a serious threat to the health and welfare of the pharmaceutical industry." [16]

The group, along with other drug companies, "pledged to donate $10 million" to add to
the previously-raised $8.6 million to battle the
ballot, and threatened "retaliatory initiatives
aimed at trial lawyers and unions" that were
most likely to support the measure. [16]

The powerful lobbying group represents forty-
eight drug companies and has a record, according to the watchdog collaborative SourceWatch, of
hiding it's lobbying activities and paying influential
organizations for their advocacy. [16]

For instance, the AARP Bulletin reported in
2000 that a tax record review showed "that
three organizations that claim to speak for older
Americans are in fact heavily bankrolled by the
pharmaceutical industry." [16]

PhRMA also spends a portion of profits
on "aggressive public relations campaigns" to
spread messages to the public about their good
works and counteract doubts about pricing,
safety and over-marketing of drugs in the US. [16]

Drug Ads

The proliferation of drug ads in American media
is a serious issue. Dr. Sidney M. Wolfe of the
Public Citizen Health Research Group says that
the public tends to think that the "FDA reviews

all ads before they are releases and allows only the safest and most effective drugs to be promoted directly to the public." [10]

In fact, the FDA only reviews a small number of drug ads and does so only on a voluntary basis. [6] Drug companies do not require FDA approval for direct-to-consumer ads. [6] The FDA can issue warnings to companies if they become aware of deceptive or misleading ads but in 2007 it issued only two such letters. [6]

Director of Health Care for the U.S. General Accounting Office Marcia Crosse said that the policing slowed after a policy was implemented to route letters through the FDA's chief counsel office, delaying the warnings up to six months. [6] "The effectiveness of the FDA in halting [false and deceptive] advertising is limited," she said. [6]

In 2005, PhRMA lobbyists said that they were developing a voluntary code of conduct for their drug advertisements. [16] *The New York Times* reported that this code was likely meant to fend off federal regulation. [16] One marketing executive said: "Better to self-regulate than to have someone else tell you how to conduct your business." [16]

Drug Research and Approval

One of the most troubling misconceptions Americans have about drugs is that the FDA does the research on new medications and that, if they're on the market—they're safe.

The fact of the matter is: it's the drug companies that fund the research and bring it to the FDA for review. Worse yet, pharmaceutical lobby groups influence the acts that determine changes in regulating policies and fund the FDA so that they can speed up reviews.

Most regulating agencies aren't in the compromising position of negotiating their budgets with the industries that they are supposed to regulate, says SourceWatch, but the FDA is. [16]

In the 1990's, in order to push drugs through the approval process faster; the pharmaceutical industry began paying the FDA millions in "user fees." [16] The Prescription Drug User Fee Act, legislation passed by Congress, supports payments of more than $500,000 to accompany drug applications so that the FDA can hire more reviewers to expedite the approval process. [26]

Today, these payments "now fund more than half the agency's critical drug-review process." [16] The agency and the industry "re-negotiate" these fees and how they're applied every five years which gives Big Pharma considerable leverage into the whole program. [16]

And testing? New medications are tested on select groups of individuals in most cases. [10] "Post-approval" testing is the real measure of a drug's safety: after it's released to the public. We're the guinea pigs. [10] The post-approval method depends upon reports of side effects and harmful reactions: that's when the FDA is supposed to investigate.

Unfortunately, the drug industry is able to stack the deck against these reports: acting director of the FDA's Drug Evaluation Steven Galson admitted in a *Frontline* interview that the FDA only receives a small portion of the reported adverse effects, maybe 1 in 10. [26]

He claimed that this is because the FDA doesn't have the authority to require anyone to report adverse events. [26]

Dr. Sidney Wolfe, Director of Public Citizen's Health Research Group, said that a 1998 study his group sponsored interviewed FDA physicians, who admitted that the system had become lax, that the standards of safety and effectiveness had declined measurably in just 3 to 5 years. [26]

Wolfe pointed out that his organization had been trying to get legislation passed, for 30 years, requiring drug companies to provide evidence that their medication is safer or more effective than an existing drug but the acts have never passed. [26] Today, no new drug is required to compare itself to the old. [26]

Professor Michael Palashoff worked at the FDA for 5 years. [26] In the *Frontline* report he told interviewers that the working perception at the FDA was that the drugs you were assigned to review were safe. If you said otherwise, you created a hassle. The management regularly edited his reviews for language and tone and omitted any written concerns about safety or effectiveness. [26]

How clear-cut was this? Palashoff said that he was told in no uncertain terms: "Don't write in your review that you're recommending against approval. Write that the data is unclear, you could go either way." [26]

He added, "You knew that if you found a problem and wanted to pursue it, it would take a lot of extra effort, a lot of extra meetings, a lot of extra justification for why something wouldn't be approved." [26]

Palashoff's term with the FDA ended after he questioned the safety and effectiveness of Relenza as a flu treatment. [26] After he did so, he was told that he wouldn't be allowed at any advisory meetings in the future and his review of the Tamaflu drug was canceled. [26]

"I think it was pretty well understood that if you were advocating turning a drug down—particularly if it was from a large pharmaceutical company—that wouldn't be good for your career, as far as promotions. It wouldn't be good for your career, scientifically, as far as being able to review other drugs in the future that had potential problems," Palashoff told *Frontline*. He resigned from the FDA following the incident. [26]

VP of the University of Arizona's Health Sciences division Dr. Raymond Woosley says: "I think Americans need to recognize that every time they put a pill in their mouth – especially a new pill that they've never taken before – it's an experiment." [26]

Post-approval testing is dependent upon doctor reports and they are completely voluntary. In most cases, says *Frontline*, they'll report to the drug manufacturer rather than the FDA. [26]

The trust involved in the whole process has been severely compromised. *Frontline* points out that Baycol manufacturers delayed adverse reports while aggressively marketing the drug. [26] The FDA claims that it was unaware of risks associated with the drug. [26]

The Fen Phen scandal? Cardiologist Stuart Rich says that approval and distribution of Redux occurred just as he was concluding a study that showed a strong link between high blood pressure and the use of such diet aids; Redux in particular. [26]

Rich and then-FDA reviewer Dr. Lutwak were shocked at the manufacturer's plans to pursue the market but had faith that it would never get through the FDA process. [26]

Dr. Jack Crary was one of the first doctors to send the FDA adverse reaction reports concerning the drug and wondered, why after many more reports to both the FDA and the manufacturer Wyeth, there was no talk about it. [26] It wasn't taken off the market until six months later. [26]

The "Death by Medicine" doctors report that back in 1986, a report by the US General Accounting Office "found that of the 198 drugs approved by the FDA between 1976 and 1985…102 (or 51.5%) had serious post-approval risks… including heart failure, myocardial infarction, anaphylaxis, respiratory depression and arrest, seizures, kidney and liver failure, severe blood disorders, birth defects and fetal toxicity and blindness." [10]

Chapter 3: Personalized Medicine

Personalized Medicine Throughout History,
Personalized Medicine Today

Hard-core conventional doctors may criticize mind-body medicine, point to the lack of research concerning complementary and alternative medicines (CAMs) and hail reductionist science but they are continually being proven wrong nowadays.

What medicine was first about and mostly about in human history, has been, health as it relates to a person's life, community and culture.

Personalized Medicine Throughout History

The divisions that occurred between "barbers" and surgeons, the divisions that were created between midwives and doctors, the co-opting of ancient medicine for purposes of patent rights, the attempts to discredit natural medicines and complementary therapies...this was all intended to create authority, credibility, respect and status—and monopoly—in the field of conventional medicine.

The most ancient practices of medicine involved treating the whole person: body, mind and spirit. [33] Traditional medicines, for example, are based on the idea that the body is "a microcosm of the universe, subject to the same natural laws." [33] They're about balance and the bigger picture.

Hippocrates is called the "father of modern medicine" and emphasized rationality and reason in the field of medicine. [33] His ethical considerations about the practice: working to "do no harm" and working for the benefit of the sick—not for personal gain—are the bases of the Hippocratic Oath that doctors take before they begin practicing medicine. [33]

But Hippocrates also espoused truly preventive care. He said that illness isn't just due to internal disorder but "outside influences such as climate, personal hygiene, diet and activity." [33] He believed that observation and written histories were important in understanding an individual's illness and he believed that most medical care should consist of diet and hygienic changes, that drugs and surgery should only be used rarely and as a last resort. [33] How many doctors today break, or are forced to break, the basic components of that oath?

The scientific method grabbed hold of the field of medicine during the Renaissance and this narrowing of focus has contributed to many advances in the field: the discovery of penicillin and other antibiotics, vaccines, and other drugs. [33]

The herbal remedies and natural medicines previously used (material medica) was soon co-opted and turned into the field of pharmacology. [33] Plants were analyzed for their health benefits and broken down into singular compounds. [33]

Modern medicine made doctors and scientists one. For most of human history, they were separate professions. [33]

Before the advent of modern medicine, most medical care consisted of recommendations about cleanliness, diet, exercise and lifestyle. [33] Herbal remedies and surgeries were used as well, but less often. 20th century medicine lengthened the human life span by conquering a host of major illnesses caused by outside agents such as bacteria and viruses but it's also contributed to a huge rise in conditions like cancer, diabetes and cardiovascular disease. [33]

The extreme specialization and splintering of the medical profession has generated scientific advances but at the same time, it's compromised medical treatment. Instead of your primary doctor having all the tools to treat you, one specialist or another may come up with conflicting causes of your illness. This extreme disjointedness in medicine has also eroded trust and the doctor-patient relationship. There's a lot to be said for a doctor that gives you his time rather than a multitude of tests.

An interesting bit of history lies behind the symbol of the medical profession: the staff with snakes intertwined around it. Asclepius was the half-divine son of the Greek god Apollo. [33] Apollo was known as the "bringer of and deliverer from plagues." [33] Asclepius inherited his father's healing abilities, learned herbal remedies from the centaur Chiron and became the basis of a long-lived healing cult. [33] He was associated with snakes (which are known to stand for wisdom) and had two daughters: Hygeia, who stood for health and hygiene, and Panacea, who symbolizes the cure-all. [33]

The staff of Asclepius is sometimes used as a symbol for the medical profession but strangely enough, in America it's more often interchanged with the caduceus: the staff of Hermes. [33] Hermes is credited with the birth of commerce. [33]

Personalized Medicine Today

So where's personalized medicine at today? It's in our own hands, for the most part, and lives in the choices many doctors are making to opt out of managed care systems and create new vehicles for real health care. It lives in the slow acceptance of ancient medicines and a wider view of health. It comes from doctors that treat the whole patient and not just the condition, and yes, advances are also being made in medicine to "personalize" drugs.

Responsibility

Jessie Gruman, president of the Center for the Advancement of Health says that the age of transparency, the advances in information technology today, has its pros and cons. [32]

Research on treatments that work reveal just how ineffective treatments in long-standing use really are; reviews of published medical studies give us more accurate information but expose competing claims and conflicts of interest; Internet information can be a valuable tool but it's used irresponsibly and deceptively as well. [32]

"Combine these with an active press, a 24-hour news cycle, the proliferation of watchdog groups, and commercial interests that manipulate scientific claims to support their aims. The result is a media environment infused with messages that tell us that our every action increases our health risks, that science is uncertain, and that healthcare professionals and institutions are not living up to their obligations," Gruman writes in the *US News* article: "Cost of Healthcare Transparency Is Trust in the American System." [33]

As trust is eroded, Gruman says, "We begin to regard all information as equal; scientific claims bear the same weight as commercial claims and are regarded with suspicion or naïve enthusiasm, depending on what suits our fancy. We can no longer sort the wheat from the chaff." [32]

Gruman says that this new transparency comes with a greater responsibility on people themselves. We must learn how to judge what we're told and when to challenge our care; we need to know more than how to pick the right website or the best information from the 1.3 billion health sources on the Internet now; we do need, she says, to become "vigilant consumers of information and services," we have to "be careful," and "question everything." [32]

That may not be the magic pill or the easy answer most people are looking for, but in the end, Gruman says, it will revolutionize our health care system and begin to restore trust in it. [33]

The power of the dollar doesn't solely rest in the hands of big business. It is the choices we make and the services we demand that's changing health care today. Instead of what the "Death by Medicine" doctors call "the extraordinarily narrow, technologically driven context in which contemporary medicine examines the human," [10] consumer awareness and demand is causing medical care to expand and consider all aspects of our lives and culture: stress, physically inactive labor, environmental toxins, processed foods and overmedication.

Thomas Goetz points out that a 2001 survey published in *The American Journal of Preventive Medicine* found that only 3% of Americans engaged in the four most basic healthy habits: not smoking, keeping at a healthy weight, not drinking heavily and getting regular exercise. [34]

That means 97% of us don't practice basic preventive medicine. *We don't take charge of the most important factors in our own health.*

Goetz believes that this may be because we don't feel that we are in control of our health or believe that what we do on our own matters as much as what our health care system does for us. He thinks that the intimidating and unpleasant aspects of dealing with our health care system causes us to become overwhelmed and disengage, leaving our health in the hands of others. [34]

But control matters and quite a bit. The Whitehall study that Dr. Marmot was involved in provided evidence that a sense of control improves health and a perceived lack of control significantly degrades it. [34]

The 2000 study: "The Impact of Patient-Centered Care on Outcomes," found that when people are actively engaged in their own health care and not passive patients, they improved better and faster, required 50% less diagnostic tests and referral and were of sounder emotional health two months later. [34] The real key, the authors found, was establishing "common ground" with their doctors.

Increasing Convenience

Convenience and real health are merging, says Goetz. [4] He points to applications for iPhones that track what you eat: calculating calories and nutritional values and advising you as far as your weight loss goals; EPSS, the Electronic Preventive Service Selector that uses your personal data to recommend screening tests; [4] and the evolution of drug information labels that we can actually read and understand. [3]

Goetz writes about the Hawthorne Effect, in which researchers discovered that when people are aware that someone is observing them, they work harder and perform better. [3] The Hawthorne Effect doesn't just apply to research studies or the real attention of a medical practitioner; it also applies to our own attention to our own selves. Just plugging data into apps like Goetz mentioned causes people to really pay attention to what they eat and how much they exercise and triggers better choices. [3]

Systems for personal health records (PHR) are emerging and the studies are being done to improve the quality of health information on the Internet.

The "Federal Research Public Access Act" or FRPAA was on the 2010 Legislative Agenda. [37] It was amended and passed, so the NIH site PubMed won't be one of the only free source of published research. Today, sites that charge subscription fees to view published research are proliferating madly. The FRPAA will require that the results of tens of billions of taxpayer dollars spent every year in research will be freely accessible through eleven federal agencies and departments. [37] This open access is meant to "ensure transparency in government and access to government information." [37]

There are a number of tools available to health consumers today, including information on how to read health statistics, tips on how to evaluate health information and guidelines for making informed decisions about your health care.

Biotechnology and Pharmaceutical Trends in Personalizing Medicine

Drug are often created and prescribed in a one-size-fits-all perspective but scientists have long known that each person's chemical and genetic makeup, the condition of their organs, the quality of and the rate at which they metabolize different compounds all affect how well (or how badly) a drug will work in any one person.

The drug industry's profit mentality has included making general types of medicines that will treat the most people but as Dartmouth University's Jennifer Durgin wrote, the result is: "undertreated, overtreated and sometimes, endangered patients." [39]

The NIH reports that: [38]

- Almost 3 million Americans are at risk for overdose when given the standard dosage of anticoagulants

- Prescription painkillers can have absolutely no effect in some people

- The effectiveness of allergy and asthma medications vary widely among individuals

As we've said earlier, *we are the experiment* when it comes to drugs approved for the market.

Pharmacogenomics is the study of how our genes affect our response to medications. [38] The goal of this research is to tailor drugs to people's unique genetic make-ups.

Dr. Howard L. McLeod, for instance, has found specific genetic markers that can help a doctor predict if cancer medications might turn out to be toxic for a specific person. [38] Dr. Stephen Liggett has found a single genetic difference in people that determines how well they will respond to beta blockers. [38] Researchers have discovered gene variations that affect reaction to asthma medications and are working to understand the varying reactions people have to psychotropic medications. [38]

Although McLeod says "Patients will have more of a say in their therapy. It'll be their genes guiding decisions": others worry that genetic information like this will be easily exploitable. [39]

The pharmaceutical industry has already begun lobbying for control over such drugs and is in fierce combat with the biotechnology industry.

The other problem with this (other than the fact that we're looking for magic bullets again) is that scientists also know that a wide variety of factors influence the expression of genes. We are not just our genes. Environmental toxins, family environment and learned habits, ways of thinking and acting...all of these things affect how any one of our genes acts in the real world. And furthermore, all of these things can contribute to changing genetic makeup over time: this is the basis of evolution: environment-gene-environment-gene. Controlling the genetic environment too closely can limit the survival of the species.

Chapter 4: Health Literacy

The Informed Patient, Tools for Taking Charge

Taking Control

Thomas Goetz says that even though all of this responsibility and taking charge of our own health care can seem overwhelming, it's best to start with three simple principles: [34]

1)   Engage

There's a lot of pressure on us to take for granted the information we get from newscasters or doctors and "leave the science to the experts." But you can question why your doctor is prescribing what he does; you can have the results of tests sent to you rather than a lab; you can go to a credible website to investigate your condition. Simply deciding to act engages something deep within you.

2)   **Be Proactive**

Goetz says that we all have health issues we ignore until they get bad enough for us to do something. We end up letting the condition control us rather than controlling the condition.

He recommends choosing a couple of things we know we need to address, such as losing weight or finding out more about nagging indigestion, and then listing two or three simple actions you could take: choosing a healthier afternoon snack every day, taking two walks every week or finding out more about your problem, either through the Internet or a specialist.

Make a start; make a list and then act

3)   **Set Guidelines Not a Regime**

Goetz reminds us that perfection isn't the goal. Even if we do absolutely everything that we can right; this doesn't mean we won't experience a health problem. It's a set-up for failure if you don't allow yourself to splurge here and there, if you don't skip the workout when you want to, if you judge yourself too harshly.

The idea is to improve your activity level and your engagement in your own life.

Any attention you pay will increase your odds of better health outcomes.

Goetz also give some basic advice for making better health decisions: [42]

1)   Know Your Options

Surgery or radiation aren't the only treatment plans available for men with prostate cancer yet most of the men that are following Dr. Dean Ormish's diet and exercise program didn't know that when they were first diagnosed.

"I heard about this group and realized there was a third option," one man told Goetz. "There were behaviors that might reduce the chances that this cancer would kill us, without surgery or radiation. This idea that there was a third choice, another path, was completely unexpected."

Goetz stresses that there are many choices available to all of us. We don't have to take the options that are handed to us as the be-all and end-all: we just have to learn where and how to look.

2)   Demand Relevant Information

There are so many health scares and statistics out there but Goetz stresses that there's a big gap "between research and relevance, between what a study means and what it means *for you*."

Just because you hear that most Americans don't get enough vitamin D, that doesn't mean you should rush out and get supplements—that could even be *unhealthy* in some cases.

Whether your doctor is talking about a new medication or risk factors for a condition, beware of generalities.

3)   Making Decisions Improves Health

Even if you are suffering from a life-threatening illness; passivity won't help you, putting yourself in someone else's hands and trusting them to make the right decisions for you isn't healthy.

Goetz points out that in the emerging model of medicine, that of personalized health, you should be involved in all the decisions concerning your care. Multiples studies have found that patient participation improves health outcomes.

4)   Small Decisions Matter

Health care starts at home, Goetz reminds us. It's the small actions we take, the "micro-choices" we employ in our everyday lives that can add up to the biggest health benefits.

5)   The Best Decision

Goetz points out that a good decision and the best decision can be two very different things. In medicine, a good decision is one that leads to the best outcome medically. In personalized health care, the best decision is the one that draws on all of the available and relevant information and is consistent with how we want to live our lives: it gives us the best quality of life according to *our own considerations.*

What is health literacy?

Health literacy is "the degree to which individuals have the capacity to obtain, process and understand basic health information and services needed to make appropriate health decisions." [40]

AHIMA (American Health Information Management Association) says that health literacy is not as simple as understanding what kind of medical provider to see or understanding what screenings to have and it doesn't have to relate to one's ability to read. [40]

Today, health literacy means: [40]

- understanding prescription medications
- being able to calculate doses
- knowing how to access medical records
- knowing how to interpret test results
- being able to read graphs
- understanding discharge instructions
- understanding consent forms
- knowing how to schedule appointments
- knowing how to request information
- knowing how to use a computer or having help to do so
- knowing how to navigate complex health organizations for relevant services in multiple locations
- knowing how to locate specialists

Low levels of health literacy costs the US $240 billion a year. [41] Why?

Chronic conditions are the most costly drain on the health care system and affect many people. Chronic conditions accounts for 75% of our nation's health care bill and 15% of American adults have at least one chronic condition. [41]

It's estimated that 90 million Americans have problems understanding health information, an issue that affect their ability to follow a treatment program correctly, keep up with appointments and take prescriptions properly. [41] People that don't understand their own health will often disregard lifestyle changes and discharge instructions. [41]

The American Medical Association (AMA) says that health literacy is a stronger predictor of a person's health than age, education, employment or race. [40]

As the use of electronic health records blooms in health care today; the ability of Americans to read, understand and manage their own medical records hasn't kept up. [41]

Fortunately, a vast array of tools is sprouting up to help us all become involved in personalized medicine.

Tools for Increasing Your Health Literacy

The Internet offers many options for managing your health care but there are a number of basic tools that will help you make better use of the Internet and your health care.

Communication

Getting the most out of your doctor's visit takes some guidance and skill. Even though all of us have been in a doctor's office at one time or another; communicating well there doesn't come naturally.

"Coached care" is the result of health researcher Sherri Kaplan's work and teaches people how to communicate effectively in the doctor's office and get the information that they need to know. [43]

She points out that when we go to see the doctor, we're often nervous, intimidated, undressed and vulnerable. Even though we go in with some general ideas of questions we want to ask; we're easily derailed. [43]

Kaplan says there is a waiting room window in which patients can learn how to focus on getting the best and most information from their visit. [43] She and her colleagues used the time a patient usually spends reading a magazine to go over their medical records with them, guide them through management possibilities and sharpened up their questions. [43]

Kaplan also told people that they needed to be prepared, needed to think of the three things that they wanted to get out of the encounter but to be flexible as well, stay in the moment and in the flow of the conversation. [43]

Communications specialist Richard Street Jr. agrees: "Medical care is a conversation. So to have influence in that conversation you have to speak up." [43]

Dr. Francesca Dwamena says that even though some people might go overboard, effective communication is a boon to both doctors and patients. [43]

"If you have 15 minutes and the patient expects to cover 20 complaints, it's pretty frustrating but I am happy when a patient comes in and has read some information about their illness and has some questions. You feel stimulated, you are on your guard and you are more careful," she says. [43]

One of Dwamena's coached patients found that although her doctor said he had only 10 minutes; he spent a half hour with her and answered all of her questions. [43]

"The doctor was more open because *she was*," says Dwamena. [4]

Kaplan says, "Doctors will tell you about the difficult patient, the patient who was obnoxious and scooped up all the time, but that's the rare exception. Most people sit there like wallpaper." [43]

Street says that during any medical visit, there are actually two experts in the room. [43] A doctor might know a lot about breast exams but a woman knows the unique composition and peculiarities of her own breasts. [43]

The point is, Street says, is that doctors and patients have to come to a consensus about what treatment will be: it's not helpful for the patient to simply accept a prognosis or a prescription. [43] This agreement has to consider "the patient's values and everyday realities." [43]

"You get very little adherence to doctor's recommendations when you didn't get the patient's buy-in on what will work for them," he says. "A doctor may come up with a diet that says eat this, this and this but different cultural groups, different backgrounds have different kinds of cuisine, things they eat and like to eat. So rather than saying 'Eat half a cup of rice,' maybe it ought to be something like 'Let's talk about what starches we can use.'" [4]

The doctor-question checklists on many health websites aren't really enough, adds Dwamena. [43]

"Patients who've been 'activated' with a checklist or other tools are actually less satisfied with their medical encounter—this is a possible explanation—because they know how things should go but they don't have the skills to achieve that goal." [43]

At the University of Michigan, Dwamena and her colleagues have developed a three-session course to coach Medicaid members on how to communicate effectively with their doctors. [43]

Role-playing and videos are used, as well as teaching patients how to tell a story. [43]

"We taught them every story has three parts: bio-psycho-social," Dwamena explains. "The physician needs to get the whole picture. The first is the physical part, which is the symptom that they came with. There is also the personal, social context of the physical problem. Patients need to ask themselves, 'Are the circumstances of my life affecting the symptoms of this disease?'" [43]

Emotions are significant too. One of the participants explained, "If I'm feeling depressed, knowing that might help my doctor. Telling him what I'm going through, what's going on in my life stress-wise, that could help him pinpoint maybe what's going on with me. I never knew that." [43]

Kaplan's work resulted in improvements in some signifiers of health like blood sugar levels and blood pressure. "We hypothesize that people who are more effective during office visits are more committed to following through on the regimen they end up negotiating with the doctor." [43]

Dr. Ingrid Taylor has created a workbook called "My Health Companion." [41] A member of Allies in Healthcare, a website devoted to providing both doctors and patients with tools to improve health care, the workbook helps people to learn to write down information during an appointment, defines medical terms and teaches people to become more assertive in communication at their medical visit. [41]

Kaplan thinks that insurance companies will soon invest in "effective patienthood" training. [43]

"If prepared patients go and use health care services more efficiently and effectively, if they follow through on doctor's recommendations more, why wouldn't insurance companies pay to make patients more prepared? Otherwise services are wasted and payers are going to end up paying for more visits because patients have goofed up their health care regimens." [43]

The Drug Facts Box

Even though the inserts that come with medications are loaded with fine print and often pages long, they really don't contain relevant information in most cases, say Dartmouth Institute researchers Lisa Schwartz, Steven Woloshin and H. Gilbert Welch. [44]

They've developed a tool called the "drug facts box" and are working with the FDA to implement it. [44]

The drug facts box lists the facts about a drug in a way that is relevant to the user.

The researchers studied the package insert for the sleep aid Lunesta and the breast cancer preventative Tamoxifen. [45]

The Dartmouth scientists say that nowhere in all the fine print on a Lunesta insert do you get any "benefits data." [45] The advertisement on the box suggests that Lunesta can help you to get 8 hours of sleep but if you look at the real data, Woloshin says, "you fall asleep 15 minutes faster and sleep 37 minutes longer than with a placebo." [45]

The laundry list of side effects, says the researchers, aren't listed in a way that makes sense: which are serious or which are just bothersome, which are more common or which occur with a placebo as well. [45]

Their re-make of the insert includes a top, middle and bottom. [45] The top part of the box

describes what the drug is intended to do, who
should consider taking it, and what kind of mon-
itoring is in order. The middle part of the drug
facts box consists of a table with research data
listing the benefits and side effects as compared to a placebo. The bottom of the insert is
the FDA approval date. [45]

Here is an example of the Lunesta Drug
Facts Box: [46]

LUNESTA (compared to sugar pill) to reduce current symptoms for adults with insomnia

What is this drug for?	To make it easier to fall or to stay asleep
Who might consider taking it?	Adults age 18 and older with insomnia for at least 1 month
Recommended monitoring	No blood tests, watch out for abnormal behavior

| **Other things to consider doing** | Reduce caffeine intake (especially at night), increase exercise, establish regular bedtime, avoid daytime naps |

LUNESTA STUDY FINDINGS

788 healthy adults with insomnia for at least 1 month – sleeping less than 6.5 hours per night and/or taking more than 30 minutes to fall asleep– were given LUNESTA or a sugar pill nightly for 6 months. Here's what happened:

What difference did LUNESTA make?	People given a sugar pill	People given LUNESTA (3 mg each night)
Did LUNESTA help?		

LUNESTA users fell asleep faster (15 minutes faster due to drug)	45 minutes to fall asleep	30 minutes to fall asleep
LUNESTA users slept longer (37 minutes longer due to drug)	5 hours 45 minutes	6 hours 22 minutes
Did LUNESTA have side effects? Life threatening side effects No difference between LUNESTA and a sugar pill	None observed	None observed

Symptom side effects		
More had unpleasant taste in their mouth (additional 20% due to drug)	6% 6 in 100	26% 26 in 100
More had dizziness (additional 7% due to drug)	3% 3 in 100	10% 10 in 100
More had drowsiness (additional 6% due to drug)	3% 3 in 100	9% 9 in 100
More had dry mouth (additional 5% due to drug)	2% 2 in 100	7% 7 in 100
More had nausea (additional 5% due to drug)	6% 6 in 100	11% 11 in 100

How long has the drug been in use?

Lunesta was approved by FDA in 2005. As with all new drugs we simply don't know how its safety record will hold up over time. In general, if there are unforeseen, serious drug side effects, they emerge after the drug is on the market (when a large enough number of people have used the drug).

The Dartmouth scientists re-made the tamoxifen insert and tested 274 people on their overall understanding about the drug. [45]

- 89% were able to correctly determine what percentage of women taking the drug developed blood clots in the study

- 71% were able to calculate the proportion and ratio of women who went on to develop breast cancer with tamoxifen and with the placebo

- Over 66% chose the better drug in scenarios that called for comparing percentages

- Half of those people with only a high school degree were able to correctly answer at least 4 of 5 questions concerning the study data

Deciphering MedSpeak

If you want to understand studies, compre-
hend your own medical records and tests
or simply read drug information and get the
gist of media information; the Medical Library
Association has a whole host of guides such
as "Deciphering Medspeak," "Medspeak Terms"
and "RX Riddles Solved!" in simple language,
moderate literacy and Spanish versions. [47]

They also offer in-depth Medspeak brochures
on breast cancer, diabetes, eye diseases, heart
diseases, HIV-AIDS and stroke. [47]

You can find their website link in our Resources
chapter along with many other useful tools.

Help in Understanding Health Statistics

Dartmouth doctors Schwartz, Woloshin and
Welch have also put together a book to help
people decipher health statistics. News media,
internet sites and even advocacy groups for
specific conditions and diseases use statistics in
alarming and misleading ways, says Schwartz.
[48] They're "trying to grab your attention by
making their disease sound as common or as
dangerous as they can." [48]

The scientists give some examples of the
problems people have with health statistics: [48]

- A drug commercial might claim that the product reduces the risk of heart attack by 50% but without qualifiers and more information; this statistic is meaningless. That number depends upon what an individual's own chances are to begin with, what their chances are without the drug, and how it might affect *them* and their chances.

- The drug might have reduced the chance of a heart attack from 20% to 10% which is very significant; it might reduce risk by 0.2%– which means that 2 in 1000 people would have a heart attack; or it might reduce risk by 0.1%, 1 in 1000 people. That's still a 50% reduction but there's only a very small risk involved.

- Bigger numbers influence people's perception more, say the researchers. A 1 in 20 chance catches people's attention more than a 1 in 10 chance even though the risk is higher with the latter. Schwartz says "We think the problem is often with how the messages are stated. Some ways of saying the same thing are much easier to understand than others."

90% of the 555 people who read a prototype of the book found it helpful. It improved statistics understanding as measured by a statistics quiz no matter the participant's educational background.

It "isn't meant to make you into a statistician or epidemiologist," says Woloshin, but to "help people understand things that can be easily confusing but don't have to be."

Evaluating Research Studies

The National Institutes of Aging (NIA) website has useful tips for sorting out alarming media messages too. [49]

Understand that there are different types of studies

There are laboratory studies, animal studies and human studies.

There are things that happen in a petri dish (in vitro=within a glass), in a living organism (in vivo=within the living) or ex vivo (within living cells but outside of a living organism). Sometimes scientists will use in vivo and ex vivo interchangeably, but of course, they're very different things.

The "evidence pyramid" below rates studies in term of their quality and prevalence and is gleaned from **Introduction to Evidence Based Medicine**. [50] Although all of the terms sound official and valid, there's a *huge* difference between a "case-report study" and a "randomized controlled trial" in terms of believability and its relevance to you.

Meta-analysis

A meta-analysis is a pain-staking and thorough review of all valid (not simply all) studies concerning a topic and a summing up of their combined findings. [50]

Systematic Review

A systematic review focuses on one kind of topic or research that answers a specific question. All sound studies are analyzed and the results summarized. [50]

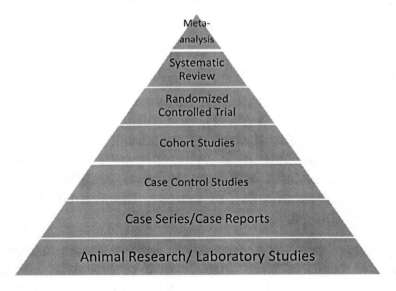

Randomized Controlled Clinical Trials

Randomized controlled clinical trials use random samples (not carefully chosen subjects that will give the results the researchers want to find) and blinding (so that neither the researcher nor the participant knows if the participant is getting the drug or the placebo—the placebo group is known as the control group). [50]

These are considered the best studies for many drugs and treatments but there are two things to consider with these types of studies: 1) they may have not controlled the environment or be of good quality according to independent reviewers and 2) some research may not use a control group or blinding or control all the complicating variables—a controlled trial, a random trial and a clinical trial are not the same thing as a true randomized controlled clinical trial.

Cohort Studies

A cohort study involves following a large population of people and comparing those with a specific condition with those that don't. These are observational studies and are not "controlled" because all of the possible factors that can affect the results aren't controlled. [50]

Case Control Studies

Case control studies use medical records and patient interviews to compare people with a specific condition to those that don't. They're less reliable than cohort studies. [50]

Case Series or Case Reports

Case series or case reports are collections of data about the treatment or status of specific patients or a single patient. They're not statistically valid. [50]

Observational or epidemiological studies are the ones most often done with people because ethical considerations hamper controlled studies with humans today. These studies often study a population of people for many years but then the effects can't be contributed to any one thing: there are so many factors that could contribute to the results. Studies that show a supplement may be helpful, for example, can't account for the fact that most people who take supplements are concerned with their health, eat better and exercise too.

Testing on humans is often difficult because many ethical guidelines (and the constant threat of lawsuits) now carefully control scientific research on humans and protect us because of grave injustices and damage done to people in the past.

Human studies are designed to bring benefit. [51] A study of people with heart disease, for example, can't compare two groups of affected people and give only one group the medication without their knowledge that this might be the case. That would be considered harmful to the group of people with heart disease that didn't get the medication.

Understand the Wording of Statistics

Like the Dartmouth researchers, NIA describes how wording can affect your perception of stated risks.

Their website describes the difference between relative risk and absolute risk. [49]

Relative risk is usually used to describe the difference between two different groups of people and is illustrated with a ratio or a percentage. [49] A relative risk might refer to the chances that medicine-receiving people have of suffering a heart attack, for instance, as compared to those that got a placebo in a study. [49]

A 1.0 finding means that the placebo group equaled the medication group in terms of risk: that means *there was no difference*. A finding of 1.5 can be extrapolated to mean that there was a 50% greater likelihood that the placebo group participants would have a heart attack. [49] This doesn't mean, however, that 50% of the placebo group *had* heart attacks. [49]

Absolute risk gives the *actual* number of problems that were prevented because of the drug. [49] If 50 heart attacks occurred in 10,000 people taking the drug and 75 heart attacks occurred in

10,000 of the placebo group, then the absolute difference in risk would be 25 per 10,000.

The NIA gives an example using bank accounts. [49] If Chris has $130, 000 in his bank account and Pat has $100, 000 in his: the relative difference could be explained as "Chris has 30% more than Pat," and the absolute difference could be reported as "Chris has 30% more than Pat." [49]

In some cases, using the relative risk sounds more impressive and in others: the absolute. You can count on a drug manufacturer to pick the most impressive-sounding numbers and choose the way to say it that will affect the most people in the way they want. They have people studying the effects of these wordings, of course.

The NIA recommends using these questions to evaluate a study: [49]

- *Was it a randomized controlled clinical trial?*

- *How many people were used in the study?* (Some studies are of only very small numbers of people and so aren't really relevant.)

- *Were the people involved in the study similar to you?* In terms of age, sex, education level, income, ethnicity and health condition?

- **Who did the research and where was it done?** A university? A government agency? Or a small, unknown lab?

- **What were the side effects?** Are they as serious as the condition?

- **Who sponsored the research?** Did a pharmaceutical company pay for it or was it funded by public tax dollars?

- **Who is reporting the results?** It's hard to trust even the most well-known news reporter nowadays. They might be getting a free trial themselves or be so overworked that they're accepting the drug company's press release and repeating the information as if they investigated it themselves.

Check out the Resources Section for other great tips and tools.

Chapter 5:
Health Information on the Internet

Pros and Cons, Research on Quality and Future Directions, Evaluating Websites

The Pew Internet and American Life Project is a long term study of all facets of Internet use in the U.S. In 2005, Pew reported that 8 in 10 Internet users in America have looked for health information online: about 95 million adults. [53]

With so many of us regularly turning to the world-wide web for information, some scientists worry about the quality of that information and what "health surfing" bodes for health care.

Pros and Cons of Internet Health Searches

In 2008, Microsoft released the results of their research, which used Windows Live Task Bar to study health-related searches on the Internet. [54] They've found that these searches often escalate into information-seeking about serious medical conditions and diseases in about one-third of the cases, behavior that could be a symptom of "cyberchondria." [54]

The researchers define cyberchondria as "the unfounded escalation of concerns about common symptomatology, based on the review of search results and literature on the Web." [55]

When Microsoft scientists surveyed Microsoft employees, they found that over half admitted that medical searches concerning serious illness interrupted their daily activities. [54]

The amount and distribution of the information and fear-provoking language increases people's tendency to become cyberchondriac. [54] The Microsoft researchers Eric Horvitz and Ryen White said the hit ratings influenced this trend: a simple search on headache pain was *just as* or *more likely* to lead a health surfer to web pages describing rare and serious conditions as it was to lead to more likely and benign causes of headache pain such as caffeine withdrawal and tension. [54]

"People tend to look at just the first couple of results. If they find 'brain tumor' or 'ALS' [Lou Gehrig's disease] that's their launching point," says Horvitz. Both researchers say "jumping to the worst possible conclusions" is basic human behavior. [54]

And this psychology is used to create key words that drive ratings that bring up the worst websites first.

Horvitz says that people tend to treat search engines as if they have the ability to answer questions like a human expert, [54] but rank results are far from adequate measures of credibility and "can lead users to believe that common symptoms are likely the result of serious illnesses." [55]

Deidre, moderator of the Health Anxiety Support website says, "People have access to medical information with no ability to filter it with a rational perspective." [59]

"Symptom surfing" reinforces unfounded beliefs, says Deidre. [59] "Bloating has about 3,062 other causes or sources, but when you are focused on your symptoms and you find one that falls in line with the subject of your investigation, it becomes simply one more 'missing link' in your puzzle. It's an affirmation of your worst fear—and a classic example of not being able to see the forest for the trees." [59]

In his own bout with hypochondria, Horvitz fell subject to the common affliction "medical schoolitis" or "second-year syndrome" in which students become convinced that they're suffering from the various conditions that they're studying. [54]

He recalls sitting at the doctor's office convinced he had a rare and incurable skin disease. He snuck a look at his chart after the examination and read: "Eric is in medical school, and he has been reading a lot." [54]

Horvitz and White say that the Pew study also found that 74% of American health-surfers don't check for indicators of quality on a website such as the date and source of the information. [55]

In 2002, Eysenbach and other researchers reviewed health evaluations from the Web and found that 70% were of low quality. [55]

In 2003, Benigeri and Pluye found that exposing surfers to health information when they don't have medical understanding puts them at risk of harm from self-diagnosis and self-treatment. [55]

Horvitz explains the fallacy of base rate neglect. [56] Certain types of evidence influence people's beliefs strongly even though the actual chances that they have a condition are very low.

"If a healthy person under 35 has chest pain, it is unlikely to be related to the heart, but because there is so much on the Web linking the two, they forget the low background probability." [56]

Availability bias also affects the likelihood of cyberchondria. This refers to the tendency people have to assume the likelihood of a serious condition simply because it pops into their head. [56] The media and the Internet make rare conditions and dangerous illnesses seem rampant and common. Horvitz says that the hundreds of frightening, serious and unlikely results that one sees on the Internet "is making first-year medical students of us all. The problem is that often, the information isn't as good." [56]

Cyberchondriac Melissa Woyechowsky explains her experience with availability bias. "I was doing these searches, and it had almost a magical aspect to it. I was on the Internet and an MS ad popped up. I thought: 'It's a sign.'" [58] This type of thinking is common in hypochondriacs: a karmic, superstitious thought pattern. One member of the Health Anxiety Support website says that even reading the word "cancer" signifies to her that she has it—or that it's on its way. [58]

One cyberchondriac says that she's received invaluable support from online groups. [58]

Therein lies the rub. Health searches aren't necessarily a bad thing and social support sites have proved to be an invaluable and health-promoting resource for many.

Horvitz and White say that health information on the Internet can affect people both positively and negatively. [55] The information can affect their decisions about contacting a medical professional, how to treat a chronic condition and their overall approach to health maintenance in unfounded and dangerous ways. [55] On the other hand, Internet information can cause people to think about their lives and make better decisions about their health, especially in terms of diet, exercise and other preventative measures. [55]

Many doctors find that the Internet can be a good source for patient education; others are horrified by the files of non-relevant printouts people come in with. [56] Dr. Pauline Brimblecombe says that the Internet has created patients "more interested in their own health and therefore more likely to look after themselves." [56]

Japanese researchers have looked at how health literacy (HL) affects health outcomes. [60] The scientists looked at diabetic's doctor visits and evaluated three levels of health literacy: functional, communicative and critical health literacy. [60]

Communicative HL is the ability to extract information from a conversation, derive meaning from different forms of communication and apply that information to changing circumstances. [60] Communicative health literacy is affected by the patient's perception of the visit and the information they receive. The researchers found that the patient's degree of health literacy affected what information the doctor gave and the patient's perception of it. [60]

How a patient perceives information affects how he or she uses and applies it and can make a great deal of difference in the management of their condition.

Another study, published in the 2009 *Community Medicine Journal*, recognized that effective communication improves the relationship between doctors and patients but wondered how patients affected that communication. [61]

The researchers studied how passive, neutral and highly-assertive questioning affected the amount of information doctors gave. [61] The patients that actively asked questions, while using sustained eye contact and positive body language, ended up with the most information and what's more, the greater amount of information wasn't just answers to their questions: they received *more* information than they asked directly about. [61]

Hopkins University's Dr. David Hungerford believes that patient's self-diagnosis and Internet misinformation derails valuable office time and compromises health care. [62] He says that doctors have to spend time clearing up patient's false perceptions and explaining the difference between hyped-up products and techniques and truly advantageous and proven practices. [62] He believes that most orthopaedic specialists feel that most Internet information is a burden and doesn't empower the patient. He advises doctors to develop their own websites or refer patients to credible websites to avoid this burden. [62]

A 2009 Korean study consisted of doctor questionnaires on the effects on the Internet on the doctor-patient relationship. [63] 89% of the physicians said that Internet information seemed to "enhance the patient's knowledge about their health," but 42.7% said that the information was often "not relevant to the patient's health condition" and 39% said that the information patients came in with was "not correct." [63]

While the general consensus was that Internet information can have a positive effect on patient outcomes, 74.5% said that Web health information made patients overly concerned about their health; 60.9% reported that this information damaged the "time efficiency of the visit"; and 56.2% said that Internet information contributed to the used of inappropriate health services, "heightening the cost of health care." [63]

Studies on Quality and Future Directions

So how good is health information on the Internet?

A 2009 study published in *The Clinical Journal of Pain* researchers rated the quality of information on websites about chronic pain. [64] The researchers entered the term "chronic pain" and rated the first 10 pages they encountered, what they guessed the average "surfer" would look at. [64] 23 websites were duplicated in the top keyword rankings and researchers analyzed 27 websites. [64] They found the majority to be poor or fair with only 2 websites meeting good or excellent quality measures. [64] The researchers concluded that "good quality information about chronic pain is unlikely to be retrieved by our patients on the Internet." [64]

In April of 2010, UK researchers reviewed Internet medical advice and concluded that it was "very variable:" 39% of the websites gave correct information about children's health conditions; 11% of 500 websites gave incorrect information; and 49% failed to answer the question that the search was conducted for. [65]

Researchers Gretchen Purcell, Petra Wilson and Tony Delamothe identified some of the problems concerning improving health care information on the Internet in the 2002 *British Medical Journal.* [66]

The researchers said that by 2002, at least 80 studies found a huge variance in Internet health information as far as accuracy, completeness and consistency. [66]

Some of the problems in setting a standard, they said, are the wide variance in types of health information: personal blogs, patient discussion groups and peer-reviewed journal articles. When people surf the net, they have differing criteria for quality: some may want simple explanations, others want hard data. [66]

But in the end, the scientists concluded, it is the surfers themselves who will define the standards and that the overall health outcomes of people have improved due to Internet use. They said that studies have also found that the popularity of a health web site often had nothing to do with standard quality criteria; consumers often find correct information without "looking for seals of approval;" and there is an "evolution from passive patients to empowered end-users who are active participants in their health care through interactions with internet-based resources." [66]

In "Untangling the Web — Patients, Doctors, and the Internet," doctors Pamela Hartzband and Jerome Groopman say that Internet access is "redefining the roles of physician and patient." [67]

The old scenario, they point out, entailed information flowing from doctor to patient with supplemental anecdotes gleaned from family and friends. [67] Today, patients can visit the same sites that inform their doctors: professional journals and guidelines set by professional associations. [67] Patients can get testimonials and advice from countless people in chatrooms and blogs. [67] Doctors themselves have more access to unbiased information.

"Information and knowledge do not equal wisdom," the authors warn, however. [67] It is doctors who can best weigh information and advise patients and doctors have to be part of the regulation and development of such information. [67]

The white paper "E-Health: Navigating The Internet For Health Information" deems the Internet "the most important, and potentially the most effective, communication medium the world has ever seen." [68] The authors say that the Internet can improve access, efficiency, effectiveness and quality of care and it can empower consumers and educate practitioners. [68]

A 2002 Harris Poll found that 90% of online users wanted the ability to communicate with their doctors online. [68] More than two-thirds of this majority wanted to be able to: ask questions when a visit wasn't necessary, refill prescriptions, schedule appointments and receive test results. [68] One-third would be willing to pay out-of-pocket for these conveniences and most said that the capability would influence their choice of both doctors and health plans. [68]

The problems the authors foresaw in 2002 were issues of legality, quality and safety, a few of the most serious being: [68]

- The traditional understanding about sharing health information has included the idea that practitioners aren't licensed to practice or share information outside of the state wherein they were given medical license.

- The twisted legal and ethical considerations about sharing personal medical information and protecting it can present quite a conundrum.

- Internet pharmacies often cause patients to skip over consultation with their doctor, and make the illegal purchase of prescription medications an easy endeavor, putting them at risk for purchasing contaminated or counterfeit medicines, outdated or wrong prescriptions, incorrect dosages and encountering possibly lethal drug interactions. [68]

In 2001, Ahmad Risk and Joan Dzenowagis looked at 13 initiatives that had been launched to improve and standardize health information on the Internet. [69]

At that time, the authors pointed out that plugging the word "health" into a common search engine like Google generated over 60 million pages [today it generates over 1 billion pages] and hundreds of thousands of health-related websites. [69]

While this phenomenon has contributed to shifts in power in all "health care actors", it can cause health harm because of: [69]

- Language and complexity barriers

- Inappropriate audience or context

- Unavailability of certain services or products in different parts of the world

- Difficulty in interpreting scientific data

- Accuracy and currency of information

- Potential for source bias, source distortion and self-serving information

Risk and Dzenowagis reviewed:

- eHealth Code of Ethics

- Health Internet Ethics (Hi-Ethics)

- URAC Health Web Site Accreditation Program

- MedPICS Certification and Rating of Trustworthy and Assessed Health Information on the Net (MedCERTAIN)

- TNO Quality Medical Information and Communication (QMIC)

- HON Code

- EC (European Community) Quality Criteria for Health-related Websites

- Organizing Medical Networked Information (OMNI)

- DISCERN

- American Medical Association (AMA): Guidelines for Medical and Health Information Sites on the Internet: Principles Governing AMA Web Sites

- British Healthcare Internet Association (BHIA): Quality Standards for Medical Publishing on the Web

- The Health Summit Working Group-Criteria for Assessing the Quality of Health Information on the Internet: IQ Tool (HSWG IQ Tool)

- The International Federation of Pharmaceutical Manufacturers Associations (IFPMA) Code of Marketing

The researchers came to 10 conclusions that they used to make recommendations to the World Health Organization (WHO) (whom they believe should develop and oversee international regulation and standardization of health information on the Internet.) [69]

1) Codes of conduct or ethics, 3rd-party certifications and a tool-based quality evaluation were key components of quality initiatives to improve health care information on the Internet.

2) A successful program should have a set of quality criteria; active, educated and interested citizens; and credible enforcement agencies.

3) Issues that were important to bridge quality gaps were the "excessive burdens placed upon citizens and the cost of implementing credible programs" with accreditation and enforcement.

4) Further research is needed to untangle the complexities involved and clarify how to improve systems.

5) There is an urgent need to include citizens of developing nations and people with poor or limited access to information.

6) The "pseudo-health sector" has no quality oversight and will likely remain that way.

7) Alternative and complementary medicine have a legitimate place in health care.

8) Language is the major obstacle in information dissemination and citizen education.

9) Coordination and harmonization are key to quality control and include all players from citizens and industry to foundations and government bodies.

10) The authors identified the following faulty concerns many have about regulation of health information on the Internet and believe that strategies must be developed to address or correct these concerns, unite stakeholders and protect citizens from harm:

- Users are ambivalent or indifferent about quality through ignorance, lack of caring, or low priority

- Quality programs that are not rigorously enforced and validated might produce a false sense of security

- Traditional media did not require quality standards; therefore neither should the new media

- Brand loyalty is more important than quality seals; the Internet has no center; therefore, it does not need central control; and, kitemarking (referring to the application of a kite-shaped mark granted for use on goods approved for use by the British Standards Institution) the Internet is like "kitemarking the west wind"

- Freedom of speech

- Free market forces

- The enormous practical and logistical difficulties associated with implementing quality programs are a barrier to implementation

Risk and Dzenowagis believe that "health information is too important to be left to the anarchy of the Internet or the vagaries of the free market, or to be conducted in a haphazard uncoordinated way." [69]

They believe that credible, global and trusted leadership is needed.

Since then, some of these players have been working to improve Internet information for consumers.

Horvitz says of the health-surfing trend, "It's an extraordinary resource for healthcare information. We're talking about a stone with a rough edge here, not a fatal flaw." [56]

The Microsoft study was intended to provide research for making the search engine better. [54] Research is underway to create smarter search engines that can detect medical queries and route people to proper websites. [54]

The Health on the Net Foundation (HON) has improved their service since Risk and Dzenowagis' review. [56] Their code of conduct applies to 6,500 health sites that agree to display information in a responsible way and inform readers about the websites purposes and sources. [56]

HON also runs Medhunt, a search engine that gathers results from only trusted websites. [56] They too, are working on building a filter that people can use with common search engines to screen information in the same way. [56]

Guidelines for Evaluating Health Information on the Internet

Guidelines for evaluating information on the Internet and the credibility of health websites have been created by a variety of credible organizations: the National Institutes of Health, the Federal Trade Commission and the Food and Drug Administration are just a few.

Evaluating Health Websites

The following guidelines are adapted from NIH's Medline Plus and the National Cancer Institute. 70, 71, 72

1) Consider the Source

Who runs the website? An individual? A business? A non-profit? A government agency? There should be an "About Us" page that tells you who runs the website and why. There should also be a valid and usable (try it to see if it actually works) option for contacting the webmaster or organization: if there isn't, it's likely that the information isn't valid.

2) Beware of Bias

The website should also say who provides funding for the site: a clue to its purpose. Is the website paid for by donations or commercial advertising? Is it publicly funded or paid for by a pharmaceutical association?

Industries with vested interest in swaying consumer opinion often create organizations and research agencies with credible-sounding names and many government agencies and national organizations also receive much of their funding from corporate industries. It isn't always evident, from the information listed on a website, to determine who really influences what is said.

According to the Center for Science in the Public Interest's (CSPI's) Integrity in Science Project, there is a long list of organizations we consider trustworthy that get much of their funding from corporations. The "Non-Profit Organizations with Ties to Industry" lists funding sources for agencies from the American College of Cardiology to the Society for Women's Health Research. [73]

The National Sleep Foundation (NSF), for instance, whose report statistics have made multiple major news headlines, claims to be "a charitable, educational and scientific not-for-profit organization...dedicated to improving sleep health and safety through education, public awareness and advocacy." [74]

NSF reports that it "relies on grants, sponsorships, memberships and other contributions." [74]

CSPI lists 16 corporate sponsors of NSF programs and says that *The Washington Post* reported that they've taken money from the makers of the sleep aid Ambien to "alert people about an insomnia 'public health crisis' as part of a marketing campaign." [74]

The Asthma and Allergy Foundation of America? 72% of their revenue in 2000 came from "corporate and other" sources including almost $500,000 from Aventis Pharmaceuticals, almost

$300,000 from Merck, Proctor & Gamble and SC Johnson & Sons, almost $285,000 from other various pharmaceutical and other industries with vested interests. [74]

You can find the "Non-Profit Organizations With Ties to Industry" link in our Resources Chapter.

3) Look for Evidence

What type of evidence does the website offer for the opinions endorsed? Are they patient testimonials? Even though many people find these compelling, they're often written by paid writers. If the testimonials are valid, there should be real contact information, not "Jane—Des Moines, Idaho."

Is the research cited marked with titles, the research organization name or the publications they were printed in or do they use general terms such as "Research studies find..."?

Does the website list the sources they've used or have they simply copied the information second-hand from other websites?

Is it clear which statements are a matter of opinion and which are "evidence-based"?

Is information given that helps you to identify the credentials of the person giving the health advice? Dr. Sue may not be a real doctor at all.

4) How Current is the Evidence?

Look at the dates used on both the article and the studies. Scientific positions change with every new valid study that emerges. Make sure the view you're reading is the most current one.

Try clicking on some of the study or source links to see if they work. If not, the site isn't kept up-to-date.

5) What Are the Website's Conditions for Quality Information?

A credible site will have an editorial review board that double-checks the information that is posted. It's good to check out who these editors are, however, since "a site on osteoporosis whose medical advisory board is composed of attorneys and accountants is not medically authoritative."

If the website has an "About Our Writers" section, check out the writers and what kind of work they've done before.

6) What's the language like?

Web writing is different than print. Bolding, white space, color and other methods are used to make information easier to glean but take a careful look: is there excessive bolding, exclamation marks, capitalization and incredible health claims? Does it make promises that seem too good to be true? Is the medical language purposely obscure and used just to give an impression of credibility?

"Breakthrough," "Cure," "Secret Ingredient" and "What Doctors Don't Want You to Know" are all sensationalist ploys used to pull unwary consumers in.

7) What's the Privacy Policy?

If you need to become a member to view content: check out the privacy policy and read the wording carefully. Do they share your information with companies "in order to provide you with useful products?" How much personal information is required? What do they do with your information? Are they collecting anonymous data to help generate important statistics? Are they giving it to interested industries?

If you're joining a patient forum or chat board: who moderates it and how?

8) What kind of links does the website provide?

Some websites are riddled with links; others have only a select few. Are the links tailored to make you buy a certain product or visit only sites of commercial interest?

Does the website have links that allow you to check data or are they all advertisements?

Do research links go to a drug or supplement manufacturer's site or a credible journal?

9) Get a Second Opinion

Just as it's advisable for you to get a second opinion from a doctor; it's important to get second opinions about the health information you've found on the Internet. In some cases, you might just want a third, fourth and fifth opinion.

Just because there are 200 websites all claiming that this "superfood" is the new breakthrough or that "newly recognized and commonly misdiagnosed condition" is affecting people all over the country; that doesn't mean that any of them are using any real evidence to back their claims or that any of them can be considered credible sources. On the Internet, prevalence does not equal validity. It just means many people are jumping on the bandwagon to make as much money as they can before they are found out or tracked down.

Evaluating dietary supplements and new drugs are completely different ballparks than the one for evaluating a website's credibility. People often think that because a drug is approved it must be safe or because an herb has been "used for thousands of years" it must be a safe alternative too.

These are dangerous assumptions. The FDA publishes an online fact sheet called: "Tips for the Savvy Supplement User: Making Informed Decisions and Evaluating Information" on its website and Medline Plus offers comprehensive information about drugs, the research on them and the risks and benefits.

There's a wealth of such websites listed in our Resource Section.

Chapter 6:
The Top-Rated
Health-Related Web Sites

CAPHIS is the Consumer and Patient Health Information Section of the Medical Library Association (MLA). They've ranked 100 websites by their criteria for quality: credibility, sponsorship/authorship, content, audience, currency, disclosure, purpose, links, design, interactivity, and disclaimers. [75]

The "Top Ten" Most Useful sites (not ranked in order) the MLA lists are: [75]

- Cancer.gov

- Centers for Disease Control and Prevention (CDC)

- familydoctor.org

- <u>healthfinder®</u>

- <u>HIV InSite</u>

- <u>Kidshealth®</u>

- <u>Mayo Clinic</u>

- <u>MEDEM: an information partnership of medical societies</u>

- MedlinePlus (<u>English</u> | <u>Spanish</u>)

- <u>NOAH: New York Online Access to Health</u>

The "2010 CAPHIS Top 100 List: Health Websites You Can Trust" link is available in our Resources Section. In this chapter, we thought we'd list the top sites as they are organized from the top 100 list in the following categories: General Health, Women's Health, Men's Health, Parenting & Kids, Senior Health, Specific Health, For Health Professionals, Drug Information Resources and Other Useful Health Sites.

Top Websites in General Health [76]

1) Aetna Intelihealth
<u>http://www.intelihealth.com/</u>

Aetna InteliHealth was created through the collaboration of Aetna Insurance Company, Harvard Medical School and Columbia University

College of Dental Medicine. It's editorial policy states that the website "maintains absolute editorial independence from Aetna," and has plenty of interactive options.

2) The Cleveland Clinic Health Information Center
http://my.clevelandclinic.org/health/default.aspx

The Cleveland Clinic, like the Mayo Clinic, is based around a team or integrative approach to health care, summarizing the best advice from all relevant specialists. This site offers podcasts and webcasts and interactive question boards. It also offers a live chat option from 10 am to 1:30 pm, Monday through Friday.

3) Familydoctor.org
http://familydoctor.org/online/famdocen/home.html

Family doctor information is written and reviewed by members of the American Academy of Family Physicians. It has a Spanish-language option, health calculators and plenty of other interactive tools.

4) Hardin M.D.
http://www.lib.uiowa.edu/hardin/md/

Hardin MD is the creation of the University of Iowa's Hardin Library for the Health Sciences. Its difference from other sites lies in its emphasis on medical pictures.

5) healthfinder
http://www.healthfinder.gov/

Healthfinder was developed by the US Department of Health and Human Services and provides many links to other credible websites as well as a child-friendly interface. Much of the information is available in Spanish as well as English.

6) HealthLink Plus
http://www.healthlinkplus.org

The Public Library of Charlotte & Mecklenburg County in North Carolina created this health information site, available in English and Spanish. It also provides real-time access to reference librarians.

7) Mayo Clinic
http://www.mayoclinic.com/

The world-renowned Mayo Clinic uses easy-to-understand language for comprehensive health information. It has many interactive features and offers blogs and pod casts.

8) Med Help International
http://www.medhelp.org/

Med Help International requires fee-free registration and is a non-profit organization that provides information and the ability to connect with others through over 200 medical forums.

You can choose between patient forums and doctor-led boards.

9) MedicineNet.com
http://www.medicinenet.com/

WebMD owns and operates Medicine Net. It's a user-friendly and interactive web site that is edited by over 70 U.S. Board-certified doctors.

10) MedlinePlus
http://www.medlineplus.gov

Medline Plus is a NIH and NLM site that is home to over 18,000 links to "accurate and current medical information." It offers Spanish links and local resources in 18 states.

11) NetWellness
http://www.netwellness.org/default.cfm

NetWellness is a non-profit site that's been up for over 10 years. The information available has been both created and evaluated by professionals from the University of Cincinnati, Case Western Reserve University and Ohio State University. The "Ask An Expert" feature is provided by professionals from the 3 facilities that volunteer their time.

12) NOAH: New York Online Access to Health
http://www.noah-health.org

The bilingual NOAH site has "accurate, timely, relevant and unbiased" health information.

Top Websites in Women's Health [77]

1) Feminist.com Health and Sexuality Links
http://www.feminist.com/resources/links/links_health.html

This website was created by the grassroots organization Feminist.com and includes directories of service providers.

2) Hormone Foundation: Women's Health
http://www.hormone.org/public/women.cfm

The Endocrine Society created this website and offers service provider finders, clinical trials in progress and Spanish translation.

3) Infertility Health Resources
http://www.ihr.com

IHR is a clearinghouse for information on many relevant topics and issues concerning infertility as well as support group links.

4) My Pelvic Health
http://www.mypelvichealth.org/

This site was created by the American Urogynecologic Society and offers information, tools and additional resources.

5) National Women's Health Resource Center
http://www.healthywomen.org

This national clearinghouse for women's health information has links to books, national organizations and local health departments besides offering original information and links to news sources.

6) North American Menopause Society
http://www.menopause.org

This site has information for both health care providers and consumers, including ongoing research, referrals and educational materials.

7) Our Bodies Ourselves
http://www.ourbodiesourselves.org

Created by the Boston Women's Health Book Collective, this site has "both clinical and psychosocial information." It has a Spanish option and links to other resources.

8) Women's Health.gov
http://4woman.gov

This site was created by the US Department of Health and Human Services. It has Spanish options and a girl's site.

Top Websites in Men's Health [79]

1) AHRQ Men Stay Healthy at Any Age
http://www.ahrq.gov/ppip/healthymen.htm

The Agency on Health Research and Quality created this website and the information comes from the U.S. Department of Health and Human Services (HHS) and the U.S. Preventive Services Task Force. It consists of a checklist that helps men maintain their health.

2) American Academy of Family Physicians–Men's Health
http://familydoctor.org/men.xml

The information on this site is available in both English and Spanish.

3) Ask Noah About: Men's Health
http://www.noah-health.org/en/healthy/men/

The New York Academy of Medicine and the New York Public Library collaborate to produce the information on this website in both English and Spanish.

4) CDC Men's Health
http://www.cdc.gov/men/

The Centers for Disease Control and Prevention provide links to hundreds of credible articles on men's health issues and offers simple-language options.

5) MayoClinic.com-Men's Health Center
http://www.mayoclinic.com/health/mens-health/MC99999

World-renowned specialists offer simple and accurate advice on a number of health conditions and have many interactive tools.

6) MedlinePlus- Men's Health Topics
http://www.nlm.nih.gov/medlineplus/menshealth.html

The NIH and the NLM offer basic information, current research news and many links to other valid website sources.

7) Urology Health (American Urological Association)
http://www.urologyhealth.org/patientinfo/

Urology Health has extensive information about a wide variety of urological conditions affecting men.

Top Websites in Parenting &Kids [80]

1) American Academy of Pediatrics
http://www.aap.org

This site offers plenty of information on child health topics from conditions and diseases to development and safety.

2) Child & Adolescent Psychiatry – Resources for Families
http://www.aacap.org (click on Resources for Families)

This website offers links to everything from helping children deal with pop culture to dealing with disaster. It has a glossary of symptoms and conditions, resources for finding a psychiatrist and clinical trial information.

3) Dr. Greene.com
http://www.drgreene.com

Dr. Alan Greene is a Stanford University professor of pediatrics. His site offers information for both consumers and health professionals.

4) What to Expect
http://www.whattoexpect.com

The author of the popular series related to "What to Expect When You're Expecting," Heidi Murkoff, has plenty of information, chat boards and support groups for parents.

5) KidsHealth.org
http://www.kidshealth.org

KidsHealth was created by the Nemour's Foundation's Center for Children's Health and has separate sites for parents, children and teens in both English and Spanish.

6) National Institute of Child Health and Development (NICHD)
http://www.nichd.nih.gov/health

The NIH conducts their own research on children's health and families. This site also offers links to other resources.

7) Teen Health
http://www.nlm.nih.gov/medlineplus/teen-health.html

The NLM uses the Medline Plus format to present teen-relevant information on a wide variety of topics.

8) Virtual Pediatric Hospital
http://www.virtualpediatrichospital.org

University of Iowa doctors created this site and it is designed as an interactive web resource for both providers and the public.

Top Websites in Senior Health [81]

1) AARP: Health
http://aarp.org/health/

The American Association for Retired Persons has an incredible amount of relevant information and resources that are trustworthy.

2) Administration on Aging Elders & Families
http://www.aoa.gov/AoARoot/Elders_Families/index.aspx

The HHS's Administration on Aging site helps the elderly and their families quickly navigate to the information that is most relevant to them. It has plenty of information on finding benefits, caregiver support, insurance and other resources and programs.

3) AgingCare: An Online Community for Caregivers
http://www.agingcare.com/

This website provides information on health issues and financial options for aging adults and their caregivers.

4) The AGS Foundation for Health in Aging
http://www.healthinaging.org

The American Geriatrics Society Foundation site has four sections: up-to-date health information, resources for caring for the elderly at home, a physician-referral guide and a community board of stories and experiences. It also contains directories of nonprofits and government agencies that serve aging adults.

5) CDC's Health Aging
http://www.cdc.gov/aging/

The Centers for Disease Control and Prevention has the latest research information, information on aging issues, links to other relevant reports and lists of relevant organizations.

6) Centers for Medicare & Medicaid
http://www.medicare.gov/

Everything you need to know about Medicare and Medicaid.

7) The Family Caregiver Alliance
http://www.caregiver.org

This advocacy group offers information on health conditions, public policy and discussion groups in Chinese, English and Spanish.

8) FirstGov for Senior Citizens' Resources
http://www.firstgov.gov/Topics/Seniors.shtml

Extensive links for agencies, organizations, programs, tax issues, health and housing, nursing home comparisons etc. for seniors (even how to request a "Happy Birthday" greeting from the president.)

9) Geriatric Mental Health Foundation
http://www.gmhfonline.org/gmhf/

The American Association for Geriatric Psychiatry created this site to promote awareness and reduce stigma associated with the mental health of the elderly.

10) Mayo Clinic Senior Health Center
http://www.mayoclinic.com/health/senior-health/HA99999

Easy-to-read articles, links and interactive health tools are available by the world-renowned Mayo Clinic.

11) MedlinePlus Seniors' Health Issues
http://www.nlm.nih.gov/medlineplus/senior-shealthissues.html

The NLM has a host of relevant information from research to local providers for the elderly in both English and Spanish.

12) NIH Senior Health
http://nihseniorhealth.gov/

The NIH provides easy-to-understand and easily-accessible information for the aging and their caregivers at this site and has videos and spoken language options.

Top Websites in Specific Health [82]

1) Alzheimer's Association
http://www.alz.org

2) American Academy of Dermatology-Public Resource Center
http://www.aad.org/public

3) American Dental Association-Public
http://www.ada.org/public/index.asp

4) American Diabetes Association
http://www.diabetes.org/

5) American Heart Association
http://www.americanheart.org

6) American Lung Association
http://www.lungusa.org

7) Asthma and Allergy Foundation of America
http://www.aafa.org

8) Centers for Disease Control and Prevention
http://www.cdc.gov

9) Mayo Clinic – Disease and Conditions A-Z http://www.mayoclinic.com/health/DiseasesIndex/DiseasesIndex

10) National Cancer Institute
http://www.cancer.gov

11) National Digestive Diseases Information Clearinghouse
http://digestive.niddk.nih.gov/index.htm

12) National Eye Institute Health Information
http://www.nei.nih.gov/health

13) National Heart, Lung, Blood Institute
http://www.nhlbi.nih.gov/

14) National Institute of Child Health and Human Development
http://www.nichd.nih.gov/

15) National Institute on Aging
http://www.nia.nih.gov/

16) National Institute on Arthritis and Musculoskeletal and Skin Diseases
http://www.niams.nih.gov/

17) National Institute of Mental Health (NIMH) Mental Health Topics http://www.nimh.nih.gov/health/topics/index.shtml

18) National Institute of Neurological Disorders and Stroke (NINDS)
http://www.ninds.nih.gov

19) National Stroke Association
http://www.stroke.org/

20) Your Orthopaedic Connection (American Academy of Orthopaedic Surgeons)
http://orthoinfo.aaos.org/

Top Websites For Health Professionals [83]

1) BioMed Central
http://www.biomedcentral.com/home/

Free access to research articles

2) Drug Information for Health Professionals
http://druginfo.nlm.nih.gov/drugportal/jsp/drugportal/professionals.jsp

3) Entrez PubMed
http://www.ncbi.nlm.nih.gov/entrez/

Free access to government (publicly)-funded research

4) National Guideline Clearinghouse
http://www.guideline.gov

Clinical practice guidelines

5) MedScape
http://www.medscape.com/

Registration required

6) Public Library of Science
http://www.plos.org/

Top Websites: Drug Information Resources [84]

1) AIDSinfo Drug Database
http://www.aidsinfo.nih.gov/DrugsNew/Default.aspx?MenuItem=Drugs&Search=On

2) CenterWatch/Clinical Trials Listing Service
http://www.centerwatch.com/patient/drugs/drugdirectories.html

3) DailyMed-Current Medical Information
http://dailymed.nlm.nih.gov/dailymed/drugInfo.cfm?id=2115

4) Food and Drug Administration (FDA)
http://www.fda.gov

5) Longwood Herbal Task Force
http://www.longwoodherbal.org

6) Memorial Sloan Kettering Cancer Herbs, Botanicals, and Other Products
http://www.mskcc.org/mskcc/html11570.cfm

7) NLM Drug Portal
http://druginfo.nlm.nih.gov/drugportal/drug-portal.jsp

8) Needy Meds
http://www.needymeds.org

9) PDRHealth
http://www.pdrhealth.com/home/home.aspx

10) RxList-The Internet Drug Index
http://www.rxlist.com

Top Websites: Other Useful Web Sites [85]

1) AMA Doctor Finder
http://www.ama-assn.org/aps/amahg.htm

2) CenterWatch Clinical Trials Listing Service
http://www.centerwatch.com/

3) ClinicalTrials.gov
http://clinicaltrials.gov

4) eMedicine Health
http://www.emedicinehealth.com/

5) Genetics Home Reference
http://ghr.nlm.nih.gov/

6) Household Products Database
http://hpd.nlm.nih.gov/

7) Quackwatch
http://www.quackwatch.com/

More Useful Sites (from AHIMA)

The Information Therapy for Consumers
www.ixcenter.org/consumers

Advice about finding evidence-based medical information on the Internet

Judge: Web Sites for Health
www.judgehealth.org.uk/consumer_guidelines.htm

United Kingdom site with guides for searching well on the Internet for health information and how to utilize information at the doctor's office

Health Compass
www.healthcompass.org

Designed to help older people navigate the Internet for health information

Forbes and Consumer Reports
www.forbes.com/bow/b2c/section.jhtml?id=9
www.healthratings.org

"Best of the Web" lists for top health pages

The Health on the Net Foundation
www.hon.ch/HONcode

Code of conduct guidelines (HONcode) and sites with the HONcode seal

Chapter 7:
Personal Health Records

What is a Personal Health Record, Pros and Cons of PHRs, Protecting Your Information, Choosing a PHR, Rating the Quality of PHRs, Some Sample PHRs, Doctors and EMRs

What is a Personal Health Record?

Personal Health Records (PHRs) are a compilation of your disparate medical records and other health information. There are paper versions of these records but these aren't as effective as electronic alternatives for many reasons.

Nowadays, we've often seen a wide variety of doctors and specialists throughout our lives, all of whom have given us different tests and treatments, jotted down observations and noted different aspects of our health. When you go for treatment, your family physician doesn't necessarily have all of your data and you may be asked to sign release forms from this doctor or that health professional.

When it comes to personalized treatment; your complete medical record is essential. When you have control of all your medical records and have them together in one spot; you're more likely to get the treatment that is right for you. When you have a record of your life habits and health history, including your family history; it's easier for you to manage your health care.

Your doctor can easily look for possible drug interactions before he prescribes a new medication; emergency room doctors can check for allergies before they treat you; a new doctor might see overall patterns that help to resolve a long-standing condition; some PHRs enable you to keep track of insurance claims and doctors appointments along with your record. [86]

Your personal health record differs a bit from your medical record. Your medical record is kept at a provider's office (each provider having a different version) and is protected by privacy laws. You are allowed access and copies of that information. [86]

PHRs are a very new concept and most people have never heard of them or don't understand what they are. The company Health Industry Insights conducted a study in 2005 about PHRs and found that 83% of health consumers had never used a PHR and half of those people had never even heard of one. [88] When people are told what PHRs are and how they work; 60% of consumers in another 2005 study supported their use. [88]

Benefits of PHRs

PHRs are powerful tools in terms of the empowered health care consumer. A PHR can get you immediate and proper care; it can save you money and time so that routine tests don't have to be repeated; it gives *both* you and your various health care providers more insight into your personalized health and allows a whole team of diverse providers to coordinate your care. [87]

An electronic PHR allows you to easily send your medical information to specialists or other providers that you are interested in without having to go from doctor to doctor gathering information, signing consent forms and waiting for them to be processed. It saves time in that each new doctor doesn't have to schedule an appointment with you to go over your health history.

The biggest drive behind personal health records is the fact that "the more consumers know about their health, the more control they will take over it and the healthier they will be." [88]

Complications Regarding PHRs

The Health Insurance Portability and Accountability Act (HIPAA) protects your medical records in terms of privacy and use. [87] HIPPA only applies to medical records kept by health providers: not your PHR. [87] PHR's are not considered "legal" health records and so protecting your information is up to you. Some PHR products are designed to meet HIPPA standards.

In most cases, you'll have to hunt down all the pieces of medical data floating around about you one by one. [88] You'll have to sign releases, show identification and may be charged a fee for copies. [88] You may also have to wait up to 2 months to receive the information. [88]

As it is now, there isn't even an agreed-upon definition of what a PHR is among all concerned parties, a problem that's slowing the development and standardization of PHR systems. [88] Until everyone can agree, figuring out what works best has to wait.

Many companies are generating their own PHR systems and comparing them can be difficult because of the lack of consensus and standardization. These systems vary by the organization that creates them: insurance company, employer, vendor, doctor or hospital. [88]

AHIMA warns that even though there are many PHR products available now; "PHR and PHR systems are still very much works in progress." [88]

What's In a PHR? [87]

According to AHIMA, these are the components of PHRs:

- **An identification sheet:** this sheet is generated whenever you are admitted or registered with a health care provider and contains your name, address, telephone number, insurance company and policy number at that time.

- **A Problem List:** a summary of your most significant illnesses and operations

- **A Medication Record**

- **History and Physical:** this is information the doctor treating you at the time collected about major illnesses, surgeries, family health history, your health habits and current medication. It concludes with findings from the examination.

- **Progress Notes:** notes on your response to treatment and possible amendments to management of your condition made by doctors, nurses, therapists and even social workers

- **Consultation:** opinions of other health providers other than your primary care physician

- **Physician's Orders:** the treatment plan, directions and guidelines for you and other members of your health care team

- **Imaging and X-Rays:** describes findings of such procedures. Actual film is kept in radiology or other relevant departments.

- **Lab Reports:** results of blood tests, urinalysis, cultures etc. *Your health record does not usually contain your blood type, a fact you should amend.

- **Immunization Records**

- **Consent and Authorization Forms**

- **Operative Report:** describes surgeries and the names of the surgical team

- **Pathology Report:** results of tissue examination

- **Discharge Summary:** a record of your hospital stay, findings, procedures, therapies, responses to treatment, instructions etc.

- **Name of kin or emergency contacts**

- **Names and addresses of doctors, dentists and specialists**

- **Living wills and advance directives** (including organ donor authorization)

Protecting Your Information

AHIMA reports that evolving privacy laws have created confusion concerning PHRs and lists some common privacy myths. [94]

- **<u>Health information cannot be faxed – FALSE</u>**

  Your health information can be faxed but it must be done according to security policies

- **<u>E-mail cannot be used to transmit health information – FALSE</u>**

  E-mail can be used to transmit health information as long as there is a way to protect that information such as an encryption and decryption system.

- **Healthcare providers cannot leave messages for patients on answering machines or with someone who answers the telephone – FALSE**

  If you have given the OK for your doctor to leave a message with someone else; leaving a message is fine. If your answering machine identifies you as the receiver of the message; health information can be left on a machine.

- **Your name and location while in the hospital may not be given out without your consent – FALSE**

  This information is only withheld if you specifically request to have your name withheld from the directory.

- **Your healthcare provider must have your approval to disclose your personal health information to another healthcare provider – FALSE**

  If your doctor has reason to believe that you will be receiving care from another provider; he or she can share your health information.

- **Your doctor cannot discuss your care with your family members – FALSE**

  Your health care provider can share health information that is "directly relevant to the involvement of a spouse, family members, friends or other persons identified by you" regarding your care or payment for that care. Your provider can share information with others if they can "reasonably infer" that you do not object.

Avoiding Medical Identity Theft Choosing a PHR

There are many different types of PHRs on the market, reports AHIMA. [88] The medium may be paper or electronic, the format can be a desktop application or an Internet-based service and PHRs are influenced, says AHIMA, by the organization sponsoring them. [88]

PHRs differ in terms of accessibility, convenience and ease of use. [88]

Medium and Format [88]

Paper

There are ready-made forms available to create PHRs and many consumers create their own. This can be useful when encountering medical data that still isn't in electronic form. The problem with paper PHRs is that they aren't readily available unless you're carting yours around all the time and aren't easy to send to a doctor over the Internet.

Personal Computer

There are PHR programs that you can load onto your computer and either directly enter data, or scan documents and add them. You can store the information on a CD or flash drive for easy portability and you maintain total control of your information but you might not always remember to carry your data with you.

Internet

Internet-based PHR products entail creating an account with your user name and password. You can approve access to medical providers and it's useful for both routine medical and emergency situations.

Computer/Internet Hybrid

The personal computer/Internet hybrid is a model in which you retain control of your health data and transfer either all or part of it to an Internet account for use in case of emergency.

PHR Providers [88]

There are a variety of PHR sponsors available now and there will likely be more in the future. Providers differ in terms of accessibility and security. You can use a PHR product supplied by your employer, your doctor, your insurance company or by a vendor.

Employers

Employers are jumping on the PHR bandwagon because helping people to pay attention to their health drives down company health care costs and increases productivity. Employee-sponsored PHRs are usually low-cost and link to your work-provided health plan but may stay behind if you choose to leave the company.

Insurance Companies

The cost of a PHR is usually included in enrollment in your insurance plan but they may share your information in some cases, to gather statistics and information for instance, and if you change providers your PHR account may stay with the insurance company.

Health Providers

The Department of Veteran Affairs has a PHR system in place because they've long established an enviable electronic record system. These patient portals are not always "true" PHRs because some are only for viewing—not adding data. These can be useful because medical data is automatically added to the record by the provider but that doesn't mean other medical data from other sources can be easily added.

Independent or Vendors

Independent PHR products offer the most personal control and range from free services to a monthly charge in cost. Prototypes for ease of use and accessibility are still being developed.

What to Ask When Choosing a PHR [88]

AHIMA has developed a checklist of factors to consider when choosing a PHR:

1) Content

- Will the product provide a complete health history?

- Will information be automatically added from doctor's offices, insurance companies and employers?

- If information is automatically added; is the transfer secure?

- Am I able to add, correct and delete information? How?

2) Ownership and Use

- Do you (the sponsor) have any ownership or sharing rights to my information?

- Can you sell my information?

- Can I specify that my information not be shared or sold?

- Will my information be used to determine my eligibility for employment or insurance coverage and claims?

3) Access and Security

- Who has access to my information?

- Do all members of the sponsor organization have access?

- Do I have the ability to control access? Can I choose who has access?

- How is my information protected from unauthorized use?

4) Portability

- If I choose to go with another company; will I still have access to this PHR?

- Can I transfer my health information to a new sponsor? How do I do that?

5) Cost

- How much will this PHR account cost me?

- What services are included in the price?

- What services are not included in the price?

- How much will added services cost me?

Some PHR Options: Quality Ratings

We'd love to have titled this section: "The Top PHR Options" but unfortunately, determining what PHR products are the best is simply impossible right now. Because there are no agreed-upon standards (or even a definition of what a PHR is) there's nothing in place to measure a PHR product against or indices to compare one to another.

Although you may find many sites that claim to review PHRS, if you try and find out who is sponsoring these websites; you'll have a difficult time of it. It's likely that these websites are sponsored by the PHR manufacturers themselves.

There are reports available from health technology research firms if you're willing to pay for them but most of the information you'll find online about a PHR product is generated by company press releases and biased affiliates.

It's the experimental stage right now in terms of the evolution of PHRs.

Having said that, there are some preliminary accreditations you can look for: The EHNAC, the CORE and the CCHIT.

- **EHNAC**

  The Electronic Healthcare Network Accreditation Commission (EHNAC) is an industry-based accreditation organization. It awards accreditation in "industry-established" standards of confidentiality and privacy, service and availability, data integrity and efficiency. [101]

EHNAC accreditations vary. There is the ASPAP-EHR, the HIEAP, the HNAP EN, the HNAP TA and the HNAP-70. [101]

o **ASPAP-EHR** [102]

The Application Service Provider Accreditation Program for Electronic Health Records (ASPAP-EHR) is meant to ensure that an organization meets EHNAC standards for quality in terms of handling health information in a private and secure way and technical performance.

o **HIEAP** [103]

The Health Information Exchange Accreditation Program (HIEAP) is another accreditation, a "stamp of approval" from the industry in terms of excellence in processing health data, managing and transferring health information and meeting privacy and security regulations.

o **HNAP** [104]

The Healthcare Network Accreditation Program (HNAP) includes a number of different accreditation sub-programs. An HNAP accreditation means that a company has exceeded industry-established standards for confidentiality and privacy, level of service and availability and efficiency in processing.

- **HNAP EN** [104]

  The HNAP EN accreditation applies to electronic health networks that act as clearinghouse or gateways.

- **HNAP TA** [104]

  The HNAP TPA program is intended for 3rd-party companies that manage health plans and benefits for other companies such as employers.

- **HNAP-70** [105]

  The Healthcare Network Accreditation Plus Select SAS 70 program (HNAP-70) is for companies that process healthcare transactions with a concentration on privacy, security and technical performance.

  For a list of companies that have received EHNAC accreditation (good for 2 years): visit http://www.ehnac. org/accredited-organizations.html. You'll first have to find out the name of the company that has created the

PHR product you're interested in (it's usually different than the name of the product itself.)

- **CORE** [114]

  http://www.caqh.org/CORE_organizations.php

  CORE is the Certification of Health Care Organizations run by CAQH, an alliance of health plans and health industry trades. CORE certifications are given to health clearinghouses, health plans, providers and vendors. There are Phase 1 and Phase 2 levels of endorsement.

- **CCHIT** [115]

  http://www.cchit.org/products

  The Certification Commission for Health Information Technology (CCHIT) is another certifying body for electronic health records. It has revamped its programs and re-opened for applications as of April 2010.

An Early Review

Consumer watchdog Patient Privacy Rights took a look at the websites of 5 PHR companies and issued a report card that rated them on the amount of control the patient has over information, the integrity and security of the PHR and the quality of customer service available. [106] Of the five companies (HealthVault,

Google Health, No More Clipboard, WebMD and CapMed) only No More Clipboard received an "A." [106]

The "A" was given because the company's privacy policy is simple and straightforward, only the user can upload information and access by other health care organizations is completely under the patient's control. [106]

Some PHP Samples

- **AHIMA** [107]

  http://www.myphr.com/

  The American Health Information Management Association (AHIMA) offers plenty of information on how to construct your own PHR.

- **CapMed**

  www.**capmed**.com/

  CapMed's PHR sits on your computer and saves medical records to a portable flash drive. [98] CapMed offers online PHRs, desktop PHRs, icePHR, icePHR Mobile and Personal HealthKey. [108]

  The ice PHR Mobile is a cell phone application that can retain health information for up to 10 family members for use in emergency situations. [108]

The products are available through the CapMed website or through HealthVault. [108]

- **FollowMe** [98]

   http://www.followme.com/terms.html

   Cynthia Soloman was a mother of a hydrocephalic son who was sick of the inefficiency and burden of the medical records she had to lug around and try and keep track of. Soloman developed the prototype for the FollowMe PHR.

   A PHR pioneer, FollowMe has the usual features plus an e-mail account and links to health information sources.

- **Health Trio** [109]

   http://www.healthtrio.com/phr.html

   HealthTrio offers services for businesses, managed care programs and individuals. The PHR It is a lifetime record for members and offers real-time interaction, health report cards and customization of health plans. John Hopkins HealthCare and Dossia have chosen HealthTrio and the Centers for Medicare & Medicaid Services is trying out a pilot plan along with the US Department of Defense in South Carolina.

- **iHealth Record** [110]

  http://www.ihealthrecord.org/

  The Medem company created the iHealth Record in 2005 along with the American Medical Association (AMA) and other key health organizations. It is a free service that offers online consultations, e-mail communication between doctors and patients, education programs and medication reminders. Patients control access to their information.

- **Laxor** [98]

  http://www.laxor.com/

  Laxor offers common PHR services and appointment reminders but it also utilizes personal health information managers to help patients set up and manage their PHRs and deal with doctors and other health care providers.

- **Life Sensor** [111]

  http://www.LifeSensor.com

  LifeSensor started in Germany and has a rough go of it as far as breaking into the American market. In 2007 however, the manufacturer ICW teamed up with Brown University to create a product that integrates a PHR with the patient's EMR so that it becomes a "source system" through which doctors and patients can practice preventive care.

The program will also set up capabilities for connecting with a regional health information exchange, networking with other healthcare information systems without replacing existing software.

- **MyHealthInfo** [97]
  http://myhealthinfo.com.my/

  This PHR is a Microsoft product available through MSN Health & Fitness and HealthVault. It offers interactive tools to keep track of your health metrics such as blood glucose and blood pressure levels; it allows access to lab results; posts health news and has a search engine that directs you to only credible expert sites.

- **Mi Via** [112]
  https://www.mivia.org/

  Mi VIA was developed to improve the health of Californian migrant workers by providing an electronic and portable PHR in order to better manage chronic conditions. Seasonal workers have very sporadic and transient health care.

  Mi VIA is HIPPA-compliant, offers directories of local clinics and services, is multilingual and free.

- **No More Clipboard** [113]

  http://www.nomoreclipboard.com/

  No More Clipboard was developed for Indiana University students but it is free for all users. It offers the usual PHR services along with health tracking tools and phone applications.

- **Patient Ally** [100]

  http://www.patientally.com/

  Patient Ally enables e-visits and messaging between patients and providers, provides reminder and prescription refill options and publishes report cards for providers and patient health besides offering common PHR services.

  Blue Shield of California and other leading health plans have chosen Patient Ally and it's received EHNAC accreditation and CORE endorsement. It conforms to HIPPA regulations.

- **Patient Fusion** [116]

  https://www.patientfusion.com/Security.pf/ Login?ReturnUrl=%2fHome.pf%2fOverview

  Patient Fusion, a product of Practice Fusion, is a free electronic health record for both physicians and patients. It has a doctor-patient e-mail service and real-time scheduling and prescription refills.

- **Passport MD** [117]

  http://www.passportmd.com/

  Passport MD is a PHR with MediConnect, the ability to retrieve records from providers, reminder applications, doctor-patient e-mail, wellness trackers, and education center and prescription discounts.

- **Vital Vault** [118]

  http://www.vitalvault.com/

  Doctors from St. Luke's Hospital decided to develop Vital Vault after being frustrated by medical record delays and snafus for years. It is available for $21.95 a year. Vital Vault has document scan and upload or direct electronic uploads options and the doctors hope to add X-ray and MRI image storage options.

- **WebMD PHR** [98]

  http://www.webmd.com/phr

  WebMD is a free PHR service and is known as WebMD Health Manager. There are multiple interactive services and patients can compare drug costs, download data from EKG machines or have WebMD translate complex medical codes into simple language.

- **911 Medical ID** [99]

  http://blog.911medicalid.com/

  911 MedicalID developed a card and medallion for an emergency use portable PHR. The credit-card sized product is easy to transport and the medallion is meant to be worn around your neck. It is meant to contain vital, not complete, medical data.

- **Google Health** [96]

  http://www.google.com/intl/en-US/ health/faq.html#phr

  Google Health allows you to upload documents or import them from health companies that Google Health has partnered with.   Access to your information is under your control and can be deemed read-only.   It offers 3rd party services to help manage your personal health as well as your

  records, services such as:

  o assessments of your overall health based on lab tests that you order

  o diabetes risk assessment and management

  o heart health assessments

  o emails that track your healthy habits and preventive practices o news and medical research tailored to your health profile

Google Health is a free service. Unfortunately it was discontinued in 2011.

- **HealthVault**

  HealthVault is Microsoft's contribution to improving health care. It's a platform for people to collect and store all of their information in one place. HealthVault and Google Health are not "true" PHRs: they are "personal health application platforms." [36]

  As IT analyst John Moore explains, HealthVault is platform upon which other applications can come together, a kind of ecosystem in which the consumer can pick and choose from 3rd-party applications that best suit them. [119]

  The boon to the system is it's interoperability between systems and different software applications. It also offers telemedicine options, coupling home-care medical devices to system applications. You can, for instance, connect your blood pressure monitor with the American Heart Association's tracking and charting software plus your doctor's EMR.

  Moore says there's a lot of bugs to work out such as who really controls the information? [119] If your Aetna PHR is on HealthVault and you switch companies; do you get to move that information to another PHR on HealthVault? [119]

The US Surgeon General has announced that it is collaborating with HealthVault to enhance their PHR offering, My Family Health Portrait, so that consumers can connect with medical providers. [36]

Other HealthVault applications include:

o Tools for controlling diabetes, heart disease, depression and other conditions

o Several different PHR options

o Pharmacy connections and Interaction Checkers

o Devices that monitor a person's vital signs and can signal emergency services if they fall

o An application for uploading lab test results

o TelaDoc, a system that allows you to consult immediately with a physician

o A tool for determining what exposures to environmental chemicals are dangerous for you and your family

o There's even a WebVet application

Doctors and EMRs

One of health care reform's shining stars has been the implementation of Electronic Medical Records (EMRs) on the part of health care providers but doctors have plenty of issues concerning their use.

Although EMRs could make the development of PHRs easier, doctors like Harvard internist Anne Brewster worry about the already-constrained time factor doctor's face.

Brewster recognizes that the EMR "is fundamentally an excellent idea" but "documenting electronically often takes more time than writing in a paper chart." [89] She says that e-mail portals, meant to increase doctor-patient communication, can increase time burden on already overworked doctors and points out that sitting down at the computer either to enter medical information or answer a slew of patient e-mails isn't something that doctors are compensated for in terms of pay or time-load. [89]

Brewster says the EMR can also be limiting in that she can't always use her own knowledge and skill to prescribe treatments. When she wants to order radiology tests, for instance, she must select a complaint or diagnosis from available options on an electronic list in order to do so. [89] In return, she gets a score that tells her whether the tests are justified or not for that choice and she must take further steps to "justify" her decision. "Patient cannot always fit into predetermined protocols," Brewster says, and "the EMR should be a useful tool rather than a frustration." [89]

Dr. Kevin Pho, in his 2008 *USA Today Blog*: "Why Doctors Still Balk at Electronic Medical Records," explains that financial considerations and systems riddled with bugs and problems make doctors that don't rush to EMR systems seem like the bad guys. [90]

The New England Journal of Medicine, says Pho, found that only 13% of doctors had made the transition by 2008 and explains that just upfront costs can be as high as $36,000 for a single doctor. [90] This doesn't include hiring staff to help manage the EMR or the time a doctor has to spend learning to use it. [90]

The money that EMRs are supposed to save? Doctors only see 11% of it: the rest going to health insurance companies and the government. [90]

Worse yet, says Pho, is that the systems are so new that they're "riddled with problems." [90]

Some reduce a patient encounter to "yes" or "no" questions and answers and offer no room for the countless nuances that take place in the doctor-patient relationship and affect the care and treatment of the individual. [90]

Harvard doctor Jerome Groopman says that when doctors are forced to ask patients standardized questions; this suppresses the kind of open-ended dialogue that can tell the physician so much more; it stops the kind of conversation "which can be key to making the correct diagnosis and to understanding which treatment best fits a patient's beliefs and needs." [90]

Hundreds of EMR products are on the market and since few standards exist; there isn't much likelihood that your primary physician's system will be able to communicate with the one at your hospital, or physical therapists office, or pharmacy etc. [90]

Health IT group KLAS Enterprises has found that more doctors are implementing the EMR. [92] "Part of it is people's understanding of the limited time frame to the 2011 deadline to get up and running. The psychological bubble is bursting, and there is a forced migration. This has to happen and this is the only way to do it," says a KLAS spokesperson. [92]

Nearly one-third of the doctors surveyed were replacing EHRs already in place, having to make re-investments because their systems wouldn't be viable for recently established needs. [92] 62% of those replacing their EHRs are replacing systems certified by the federally supported Certification Commission for Health Information Technology. [92]

The $19 billion that Congress has agreed to put forth to help digitize health records makes only a small dent in the estimated $150 billion total cost of meeting the 2014 deadline for the complete overhaul. [93]

Physicians and their practices can get $44,000 to $64,000 in incentives but standards still haven't been established for the secure collection and handling of the information, a serious obstacle that leaves doctors fearing privacy lawsuits. [93] The lack of standards also means that the system a doctor chooses today could not make the cut when federal measures are established. [93]

There's also the problem of paying for training. Health information researcher Ritu Agarwal says that "Study after study show that physicians in their small and medium-sized practices are extremely challenged with incorporating technology into their current flow. They haven't been able to afford it. We would anticipate seeing significant spending on training dollars...and if the government is going to help pay for that, through some pilots and demonstrations, that will help move things along." [93]

It's both unrealistic and unfair, says Pho, to put so much of the burden of digitizing the U.S. medical system on the shoulders of doctors. [90]

In April of 2010, researchers released a summary of their findings on the use of EMRs by staff at 26 small and medium medical practices for two years and their effect on communication. [91]

The doctors and staff said that:

Pros

- EMR data gave them more time to focus on patients because they didn't have to gather all of the relevant information from disparate sources ("we do not have to call down the hall for a lab or test result, we spend more quality time in a more context-rich way")

- Staff can instant message doctors during visits rather than physically interrupting a session

- Easy access to information enriches patient education; the doctor can more easily explain the how's and why's of decisions and even print out relevant information for the patient

- E-mail between doctors and patients "lowered communication barriers" and "improved the quality of the relationship"

- Real-time communication between doctors was enhanced ("I know I can now so easily and quickly give information to specialists who call.")

- The EMR enhances cohesion and team effort when doctors work together

- Showing patients their medical records increases the accuracy of that information and facilitates joint decision making

- The EMR can increase efficiency with tasks between staff that don't require face-to-face communication like scheduling follow-up visits

Cons

- The computer can be a distraction during sessions, say some doctors

- In some cases, doctors engage *less* with patients because so much information is already available ("my concern now is that we're listening less because we have more information when we walk in the room, and it's not all trustworthy.")

- Filling in checkboxes reduces open-ended questions

- Communication tools that don't synchronize together well can bog down EMR communication as far as time lags between emails and instant messages

- Communication convenience can become a habit when real-time communication is needed, such as in patient emergencies.

- Many EMR users can have "overly optimistic expectations" of data on the EMR that may have been inaccurately entered

- The reduced real-time communication between staff might reduce cohesion between them ("The best way to ensure good coordination of care is for two physicians to speak with each other directly. You can't approach any technology solution, in as complex and risky a work environment as the practice of medicine, and have it be a substitute for appropriate human interactions.")

Chapter 8:
Saving the Doctor-Patient Relationship

The Placebo Effect, Contextual Healing, Doctor Burnout, Doctor Shortages, Doctors Fighting Back

When people hear the word "placebo" they often think of sugar pills or traveling doctors as pictured in old movies: sham elixirs and quackery, but this effect is crucial to healing and makes up a large part of the doctor-patient relationship. Placebos often work as well as—and sometimes better–than conventional treatments. They've proved especially useful in managing chronic conditions like: anxiety, arthritis, asthma, chronic fatigue, digestive disorders, depression, headache, insomnia and chronic pain. [120]

Doctors are often pressured to prescribe placebo treatments from patients that come in with information from the media. The most common placebo given is antibiotics for colds. [120]

The placebo effect is such an established phenomenon that it has become a whole field of medical research in and of itself. Researchers have even found that color, cost, size and other factors of placebo medications affect outcomes. Fake surgery works better than injections; injections are more effective than pills; placebo capsules generate better results than tablets; the bigger the pill, the bigger the cost— the better they work. [123]

The more time a doctor spends with a patient, the more likely that a prescribed treatment will work. Telling someone "this will work" improves health outcomes significantly more than saying "this might help." [123]

Acupuncture has been the focus of considerable research concerning placebos. It's been proven repeatedly that acupuncture is very effective at treating irritable bowel syndrome and lower back pain. [120] Some researchers believe that this may be so because the patient receives more attention, empathy and time than they would in a conventional doctor's office today. [120] Strong evidence exists for this theory because fake acupuncture often works just as well as the real deal. [120]

The placebo effect is in the process of being re-named "contextual healing" because healing isn't just about a pill: it's "the psychosocial context that surrounds the patient:" from a doctor's attitude to the patient's social relationships. [120]

Physician Dr. Hanson says: "A lot of it is just taking the time to help the patient get a better sense of why their body is doing what its doing. It's a placebo effect in the sense that you are redirecting them in their thoughts about their health. A good therapeutic relationship helps people in and of itself." [120]

Dr. Ted Kaptchuk says it isn't even the amount of time spent. "It has more to do with being able to connect with the patient."

Mayo Clinic's Dr. Jon Tilburt says that prescriptions have become a stand-in for the true doctor-patient relationship. "Our health care system isn't really set up to reimburse for empathy; it reimburses for widgets. So doling out something becomes sort of a modest gesture toward a mutual hope that the patient will get better." [120]

Kaptchuk points out that pain and placebo studies have shown that improvements occur because of the "ritual of the clinical encounter," and that they've also found that an actual treatment isn't even necessary to create this effect. [121] This has led to the proposal he and Franklin Miller make that the placebo needs re-defining in order to shake off the negative connotation the word has. Renaming the effect "contextual healing" allows us to make use of its power and accept the mind-body influence in health. Placebos themselves are inert: healing processes occur through the mind.

Miller and Kaptchuk define contextual healing as "healing resulting from the clinical encounter...clinician-patient interaction...that aspect of healing that is produced , activated or enhanced by the context of the clinical encounter." [121]

Many factors play a role in this context the researchers say, including: "environment of the clinical setting, cognitive and affective communications of clinicians and the ritual of administering treatment." [121]

"Attention to contextual healing signifies that there is more to medicine than diagnosing disease and administering proven effective treatments. This has long been recognized under the rubric of 'the art of medicine.'" [121]

Researchers Daniel Moerman and Wayne Jonas explain that placebo study has been confounded by the fact that "One cannot...avoid meaning while engaging human beings:" there is no way to separate the placebo effect from other forms of treatment. [123] They propose re-naming the placebo effect "the meaning response." [123] "For human beings, meaning is everything that placebos are not, richly alive and powerful." [123]

Moerman and Jonas wonder why we can feel better if a doctor tells us "You'll be fine" but have such a hard time doing the same thing for ourselves and they wonder why it is that medicines are having less and less effect nowadays.[123]

They theorize "as we have clarified, routinized, and rationalized our medicine, thereby relying on the salicylates and forgetting about the more meaningful birches, willows, and wintergreen from which they came—in essence, stripping away Plato's 'charms'—we have impoverished the meaning of our medicine to a degree that it simply doesn't work as well as it might anymore." [123]

This is the idea behind "meta-placebos" or "curabo treatments." [123] A meta-placebo involves helping people to understand how the placebo effect is powerful and how they might ignite the powers of their own minds and insights to help a treatment work. [123]

Harvard professor Matthew Budd has developed an approach for doctors and patients to improve their communication in order to improve health outcomes. He developed a program known as the "Personal Health Improvement Program" and has authored the book **You Are What You Say.**

In a Hoffman Institute interview Budd explains what healing is really about: [123]

"One of the things that most people aren't aware of is that healing is a perfectly normal and natural phenomenon. When you cut your skin by accident or when a surgeon does it by intention, the surgeon may sew it up, but that isn't healing the wound. The wound heals as an expression of a natural phenomenon. Healing is natural and normal. I think that occurs not only on a physical level, healing forces also restore balance and harmony. What many of us do is impede our own healing."

"Healing is a birthright of the organism. I'm talking about the physical, emotional and relational restoration that is the relationship of intimacy; a contextual healing of harmony and trust in which a person feels at home in the world. Those things are impeded by certain barriers. An infection in a wound, the growth of bacteria, would be a barrier to physical healing. The barrier needs to be treated and removed before the healing will occur."

Budd says that barriers to healing are often things like anger, arrogance, anxiety, fear and lack of relationship. [123]

Psychologist James Kepner says that "Healing is not the curing of pathology. It is the creation of the healing context, where changes occur that could not occur before. This context is not limited to the therapeutic relationship. It must involve the survivor's support, interpersonal relationships and human environment. Healing is not just a change within the individual...[but] a challenge and reformation of the whole field." [123]

So what's happened to the doctor-patient relationship in health care today? What has happened to "the art of" medicine?

Doctor Burnout and Shortages

In 2008, The Physician's Foundation released a startling report: doctor dissatisfaction with how health care policy affects their practice will likely contribute to doctor shortages in the future. [124]

"The bottom line," said President Lou Goodman, "is that the person you've known as your family doctor could be getting ready to disappear—and there might not be a replacement." [124]

VP of the Foundation, Walker Ray, says "At a time when the new Administration and new Congress are talking about ways to expand access to healthcare, the harsh reality is that there might not be enough doctors to handle the increased number of people who might want to see them if they get health insurance. It's as if we're talking about expanding access to higher education without having enough professors to handle the influx of students. It's basic supply and demand." [124]

Doctors report that government regulation, paperwork and reimbursement difficulties keep them from "the most satisfying aspect of their job: patient relationships." [124]

The Foundation report found that: [125]

- 78% of doctors say that there is a shortage of primary care physicians today

- 94% of doctors say that non-clinical paperwork has increased in the last three years and 63% say that this paperwork is why they spend less time with each patient

- 82% of doctors say that if Medicare reimbursement cuts are made; their practice would become unsustainable

- 60% of doctors would not recommend the profession to the young

- 49% of doctors say that they plan to reduce their number of patients or stop practicing medicine altogether in the next three years

From 1995 to 1998 the Generalist Provider Research Initiative (GPRI) took a look at career satisfaction among practicing doctors. [126] The study was implemented after managed care came into being and an early survey of young doctors found that had they the choice to do it over again, 40% would not have gone to medical school. [126]

The GPRI findings included the following: [126]

- Time pressure was the strongest reason for doctor dissatisfaction

- The mental health of doctors was related to lack of control over the workplace

- Group care, as in HMO's gave some freedom from administrative burden but increased patient load

- Doctors in HMOs had lower satisfaction overall than all other models of practice

- Pediatricians reported that relationships with patients, colleagues and communities increased job satisfaction

- Rural physicians also reported that patient relationships, life in small communities and clinical autonomy were the greatest sources of satisfaction

The new health care bill is sure to increase doctor shortages. The Association of American Medical Colleges (AAMC) reports that America may be short as many as 150,000 doctors in the next 15 years. [127]

The biggest hit will be in primary care physicians, who take on the biggest role in managing a patient's total care and often are paid the least. It's estimated that there are 352,908 practicing primary care doctors right now and that we'll need 45,000 more by 2020. [127]

The problem is: medical school enrollments have declined steadily over the years and the number of students entering family practice fell by more than 25% between 2002 and 2007. [127]

And even if there were more people signing up, the other problem is, the AAMC says there will be bottlenecking because Medicare-funded residencies haven't been expanded. [127]

Ted Epperly, president of the American Academy of Family Physicians says, "It's like giving everyone free bus passes, but there are only two buses." [128]

Worse, health care reform hasn't addressed doctor needs or dissatisfaction. Specialization, marketed medicine, improper training and a host of other factors continue to haunt health care reform.

One second-year resident explains "primary care residencies are not in the sexier end. A lot of these [speciality] fields are a lot sexier to students with high debt burdens." [127]

Dr. Robert Flaherty agrees. He closed his private practice in 2005 because "I constantly felt that conflict of going faster than I should. Everyone knows if you want to make a decent living, become a specialist; if you want to be banging your head, go into primary care." [128]

Former president of the Massachusetts Medical Society John Auerbach says that people trained to intervene during a heart attack make much more than the doctor that works to prevent it in the first place. "We have devalued the work of what a primary care physician does." [128]

Epperly says that a 30% pay increase for primary care doctors would at least bring them to a salary still $100,000 less than what a specialist makes. [128]

Ob/gyn Dr. Tara Wah recently left 5,000 patients in Florida. [129] In a letter to her patients she wrote that she "could no longer afford to make ends meet," that she was "working longer hours than ever" and that "insurance payments for patient care have stayed virtually the same for the last 15 years, while the cost of doing business, including health insurance, staff salaries and supplies have risen." [129]

Wah, who no longer practices medicine, said "I feel guilty. I dream about [medicine]. I am so angry. I think, 'What a waste of my training.'" [129]

The Physician's Foundation survey found that over 10% of the 12,000 primary care doctors they talked to planned on finding a job outside of health care in the next 1 to 3 years. [129]

Dermatologist Patricia Perry is looking for an "out," sick of struggling with all of the costs and insurance reimbursements. [129] She says, "When you get to a point where you feel unappreciated and you're arguing with people about getting paid, it takes away the passion for what you do." [129]

Pediatrician Douglas Evans is considering a career change too. [129] He explains that when a teenage football player came in with a neck problem, Evans had to get authorization for an X-ray, something that can delay treatment by several days, an interim in which the boy's condition could worsen and Evans is open to a malpractice suit. [129]

Evans also says that the insurance reimbursement he gets doesn't cover the true costs of treatment. "You can't go to Wal-Mart and pay half the price for a loaf of bread and take the whole bread," he points out and says that many doctors end up absorbing the difference. [129]

In a 2009 All Things Considered interview on National Public Radio, doctors Greg Darrow and George Knaysi talk about some of the problems with our health care system. [130]

Today, family practitioner Darrow says, doctors are expected to reach a "production target" in terms of patients and pay. He says that the marketing, the quarterly numbers and all of the business aspects of medicine today interfere with its practice and that he gets fed up with having to "fulfill the hoops of the corporation." [130] He ends up wanting to say: "Leave me alone, I know what I do best, which is to take good care of people." [130]

Kynasis, a specialist in surgical oncology, has it somewhat better. "We still control our life a little bit more; there's nobody really looking at us, telling us how we should do," he said, but "we've had tremendous change in not just the scientific part of medicine and surgery, but also business." [130]

Costs of keeping the practice going keep rising while reimbursements fall, Knaysi says. "I used to joke that we were going from Nordstrom's to Wal-Mart. The big challenge is to maintain quality with high volume." [130]

Both doctors agree that increased numbers of tests and procedures are part of the reason health care costs are so high but lawsuit-fear is intense too. Knaysi says, "At the end of a 20-minute operation I've signed, dated…my name 13 times and there's a nurse who has probably cranked out maybe 10 or 15 pages of printout. We don't even look at it; it's just there in case something happens." [130]

Patient behavior drives those tests too, says Darrow. [130] He has to treat people guardedly because they come in asking for this drug or that, wondering if they have this condition or that, asking him "Don't I need a MRI?"

Doctor distress is a serious issue. Mayo Clinic researchers have found that distress greatly increases the risk of medical errors. [131] Medical residents, for instance, those that suffer from burnout, pose as much risk to patients as those that are suffering from total fatigue. [131]

Health professionals suffer from much higher rates of anxiety, depression, alcohol and drug abuse and suicide than do the normal population. [132] Doctors especially suffer from divorce and marital problems, drug and alcohol abuse and suicide. [132]

The following are symptoms of burnout: [132]

- Acting out (alcohol, drugs, extra-marital affairs, gambling, shoplifting etc)

- Apathy

- Bitterness, irritability and resentment

- Depression

- Fatigue

- Feelings of failure and guilt

- Increased chronic pain and minor illnesses

- Loss of humor or excessive black humor

- Objectifying the patient

- Poor concentration

- Reduced personal contact with patients and colleagues

- Resistance to change

- Stereotyping

- Suspicion and mistrust

- Work avoidance

Physician burnout has been linked to the feeling of "diminished control of their destiny." [132] The factors in health care today that contribute to burnout in doctors are:

- Constant reorganization

- Workload pressures

- Inadequate resources

- Inappropriate management techniques

- Role conflicts and ambiguities

- Lack of career progression

- Inadequate support

- Lack of controls

- High patient expectation

- Low patient compliance

The problems with our health care system and the doctor-patient relationship are complex, diverse and profound and the following doctors outline the issues well: Dr. Richard Friedenberg, Dr. Arnold Relman and Dr. Bernard Lown.

Dr. Richard Friedenberg [133]

Radiologist Richard Friedenberg believes that technological advances after WWII led to the splintering of medicine into specialized fields. As patients are referred out, their relationship with their primary care provider diminishes. Today, patients may see many different health providers because of the corporate and group models of practice.

This corporate development has led medicine into business, wherein profit takes precedence over the doctor-patient relationship. When insurers edged into patient management, trust in doctors began to falter. This crucial part of the healing process is consistently damaged by having to change doctors, change insurance plans and none of the "management" that occurs takes into account the idea that a patient's trust is what informs their evaluation of a doctor's knowledge or skill.

A patient is unlikely to follow through on treatment plans when their visits are rushed and their relationships with health providers are shallow.

Friedenberg says that patient satisfaction with their doctors, doctor satisfaction, respect for doctors and trust in the health care system is declining. The field of medicine is now in the age of the payor, wherein cost rules over quality and power is in the hands of bureaucrats.

Medical students aren't schooled in the doctor-patient relationship or in business management, yet today those are the core skills they'll need to succeed.

Dr. Arnold Relman [134]

Dr. Relman says that the business model of medicine is in direct contradiction to the vows doctors take.

People count on doctors to advise them altruistically, to guide them through decisions they are not informed enough to make on their own and to make choices based on the best interests of the patients.

Businessmen, on the other hand, are expected to act on their own behalf, increasing profit and not assuming responsibility for the consumer's knowledge or what is in their best interest.

In health care today, the doctor must play the double role of profit-protector and patient advisor.

The "corporatization of health care" compounds this double role. Most health care systems, whether they are clinics, hospitals, nursing homes or diagnostic labs, are owned and operated by for-profit investors. Relman estimates that one-third of non-public health facilities are investor-owned businesses and two-thirds of health maintenance organizations are part of the medical-industrial complex.

This business model has forced public health institutions to respond in the same manner, to act as competitive market members instead of philanthropic social institutions. Decisions are made according to profit considerations rather than the needs of the people; services are limited for the poor; everyone is forced to market themselves, advertise, and recruit more and more paying people.

Where self-promotion was once considered unethical for doctors to practice; it is now commonplace and essential.

Relman says that we need a health care system "that allows physicians to be advocates for their patients and rewards them for their clinical diligence, competence and compassion rather than for the over- or under-use of resources in the pursuit of profits."

Dr. Bernard Lown [135]

Lown despairs that the practice of medicine has been turned into a business and that doctors have been de-professionalized and patients de-personalized.

He says that in his 50 years of practice, he's watched medicine transform from "a healing occupation dominated by professionals" to "an industrial process run by technicians."

What is says about society is dark, Lown says, because it signals the "marketization of all human transactions." Its impact "is to denature fundamental human values and tear apart the ties that nurture communal life."

The failure of the US health system, however, affords us a look at, and an opportunity to change, the "fundamental flaws of a market-driven consumer society," Lown says.

He believes that scientific advances in medicine have freed us from common illnesses and prolonged life but at a cost: it first reduced medicine to science, reduced people to biomedical subjects and turned physicians into "super-specialized technologists." Doctors are awarded research grants not for their commitment and care, but for their mastery of science and technology.

Science also promoted disease-based care instead of patient-based care and there are powerful economic incentives to look at the doctor-patient relationship in terms of procedures instead of prevention. "Society places a far higher premium on using technology than on listening or counseling," says Lown. " A doctor earns more from performing a procedure requiring a single hour than from an entire day spent communicating with patients."

70% of practicing doctors, says Lown, are specialists: they've been trained in technical skills but have lost the "art of healing."

The science model of medicine serves the pharmaceutical industry well but not people. People are complex systems, says Lown, with cultural, economic, familial and social factors affecting the whole operation and outcomes. Listening with care, says Lown, provides insights that are "indispensable to the act of healing." Scientific-based medicine ignores this and leaves patients feeling abandoned.

Lown says that "the commodification of heath care" doesn't take social needs into account.

The "buyer beware" philosophy comes from factors such as: the consumer knows what he needs, the consumer has a choice about buying the product, the consumer has a variety of choices to choose from, the consumer has basic knowledge from which to compare products and the consumer has bargaining power.

In health care, the consumer has to have health care (they don't have bargaining power), does not understand what they need, cannot compare differences in quality, they aren't given much of an option about kinds of health care and don't know enough to manage their own health care or compare treatments.

Most of the profit from "market medicine" isn't reinvested in the community through medical education and research: the bulk goes to private investors and senior management.

"Only a wide mobilization of health professionals and patients can reclaim the soul of medicine," Lown says. "The health of a civil society is ultimately secured by interacting dependencies of people expressed in communal life."

Cookbook Medicine

Take Back Medicine member Dr. David McKalip wrote "An Open Letter to America's Physicians" in June of 2009 in which he warned that the health care reform as it stood would erode the professionalism of doctors and turn them all into technicians. [136]

He says that the Federal Coordinating Council on Comparative Effectiveness will create "quality and efficiency goals" and force doctors through a "pay for performance" model.

McKalip says that there is not one practicing physician on the council and that if a doctor chooses to prescribe treatment based upon their skill, knowledge and experience: they'll be punished. [136] And so will patients, McKalip points out. Chronic conditions, which affect health care costs so dramatically, take the most time and the most care to treat. These are the patients that doctors will be forced to avoid.

Doctors that "comply" get a rating from insurance companies and the government; doctor ratings will be lowered if they go over a set amount of cost on patient treatments. Doctors will be forced to buy an EMR to report data to the government at a total cost of $120,000 over five years. [136]

McKalip finds it incredible that more power will be given to insurance companies and the government when it was their policies that created the health care crisis to begin with.

Senators and doctors Tom Coburn and John Barrasso also take issue with the Comparative Effectiveness (CER) plan as it stands. [137] Coburn says that the best doctors tailor treatment to suit the person, using both the art and the science of medicine. [137] CER will limit doctor's ability to choose treatment and limit how much they can spend. [137]

"If we're going to go to cookbook medicine, let's just go and admit that 20 percent of the people in this country [are going to lose out]," Coburn says, while "about 80% are going to do fine. One of the reasons we have such good medicine is that we've allowed the art of medicine to flourish in this country." [137]

Barasso's criticism is that the reform centers on government instead of the patient and that there are no incentives built in to encourage people to practice healthy habits that could prevent the development of chronic diseases. [137]

The idea of "quality metrics" isn't such a bad one. After all, the Commonwealth Fund has found that inefficient and poor quality in health care costs the US $50 billion to $100 billion every year. [138]

But rushing into the pay-for-performance model without figuring out who determines quality and how that is used is a different story. A study by the Government Accountability Office said that "discretion given to managers to set performance metrics and to pay employees accordingly means these systems lack transparency and accountability." [138]

The government has funded Medicare pilot pay-for-performance programs in 260 hospitals. In one example, experts decided that blood sugar levels in diabetics had to be strictly controlled, with any elevation generating bad ratings for doctors and hospitals. [139] But just recently, a study published in *The New England Journal of Medicine* found that patients with strict blood sugar regulation died more often than patients that were on a more flexible protocol and in another study, called "ACCORD", so many patients died when their sugar levels were rigidly controlled that the research had to be abandoned. [139]

What is best for a patient isn't always the norm.

In Massachusetts, quality metrics are severely enforced. Doctors that don't comply are "publicly discredited and their patients are required to pay up to three times as much out of pocket to see them." [139]

Worse, a UCLA study has found that using the federal quality measures did not lower risk of death from heart failure and an analysis of the Medicare pay-for-performance pilot found that *complying or deviating from quality metrics had no relationship to health complications or health outcomes of patients.* [138]

Dr. David Sackett, who pioneered evidence-based medicine said "Half of what you'll learn in medical school will be shown to be either dead wrong or out of date within five years of your graduation; the trouble is that nobody can tell you which half—so the most important thing to learn is how to learn on your own." [139]

New Directions

In **Making a Killing: HMO's and the Threat to Your Health,** authors Jamie Court and Francis Smith make some recommendations on how to really revamp health care. [140]

Consumer Power

Since insurance companies are managing patient care; people should have the right to sue them (they're protected now) instead of just hostage doctors.

Doctor Autonomy

"Gag policies," those that prevent a doctor from really telling a patient what the best treatment for them would be need to be banned and treatment decisions should be made by the doctors themselves, not executives or policy makers.

Non-financial incentives need to be put into place to strengthen the doctor-patient relationship.

Justify Profits

Transparency means that everyone should know where medical profits are going and premium raises should be justified. Doctor reimbursement regulation should also be transparent.

In a letter to the Senate in 2009, the Mayo Clinic proposed, "What if instead, the system rewarded doctors and hospitals for spending time with patients, for doing a procedure successfully, for the fact that you leave the hospital without a fall or infection, and for providing excellent service to you while you were under their care?" [141]

The Mayo Clinic is the oldest and largest patient-centered and integrated care models. [142] Health practitioners of all kinds and specialties come together in a team approach to serve the patient in the best way. [142]

The clinic was founded by brothers Charles and William Mayo who insisted that doctors work on salary and practice in groups. [143]

Dr. William Mayo said, "As we grow in learning, we more justly appreciate our dependence upon each other. The sum-total of medical knowledge is now so great and wide-spread that it would be futile for one man to attempt to acquire, or for any one man to assume that he has, even a good working knowledge of any large part of the whole. The very necessities of the case are driving practitioners into cooperation. The best interest of the patient is the only interest to be considered, and in order that the sick may have the benefit of advancing knowledge, union of forces is necessary." [143]

The Mayo Clinic illustrated how the system now doesn't reward cooperation and team effort in their letter to the Senate. [141]

They told the story of an aging patient who ended up in the emergency room when he fainted. A CT scan found calcification in his heart. A stress test found an abnormality in his heart. A heart catheterization found a blocked bypass. Stents were inserted but the patient continued to faint.

When the patient came to the Mayo Clinic, a team of doctors "conducted a lengthy assessment" and determined that all the man needed was an adjustment of his medications.

Medicare paid for all of the tests and procedures performed at the first hospital but refused to pay Mayo Clinic for the office time spent with the patient.

More and more doctors are simply opting out. Dr. John Bennet, for instance, refuses to take Medicare because it interferes with the doctor-patient relationship. [144] He chooses "to continue to practice medicine according to my professional training, my professional judgment and the guidance of my God." [144]

Doctors are joining networks that provide "concierge care" or becoming part of "medical homes" in order to increase patient time, lessen bureaucratic burden and practice the "art and science" of medicine.

Nurse practitioners and physician assistants are becoming a common part of medical practice and in some cases, dominating it.

More and more, integrative medicine is the path that doctors and patients are choosing, medicine that takes the best of all fields and all practices into account.

Chapter 9:
Nurse Practitioners and
Physician's Assistants

Nurse Practitioners, Physician's Assistants and other Treatment Providers

As HMO's proliferated in the 1990's, so too did the number of patients a doctor was expected to see in a day. The gap between a doctor's available time (and the number of doctors available) and increasing patient numbers created a vacuum, a need, one that nurse practitioners (NPs) and physician's assistants (PAs) stepped in to fill.

Doctor's use of nurse practitioners and other health educators helped move medicine towards a team approach. Now, retail clinics run solely by nurse practitioners are also blooming and many people wonder about the quality of their care.

In 1996, the Columbia Advanced Practice Nurse Associates (CAPNA) opened in Manhattan. [145] In a *60 Minutes* profile about CAPNA, Morley Safer said a nurse practitioner is "a highly trained professional who is providing an alternative to the expensive primary care physician—some say a better alternative." [145]

Cost is one of the factors that has contributed to the bloom of such practices, and HMO's have been behind the push to allow nurse practitioners greater freedom to practice, but that's not the greatest impetus. Besides need, the doctor-patient relationship is often better served by nurse practitioners.

From 2004 to 2009, the number of nurse practitioners in the U.S. rose by almost 40%. [149] The American Academy of Family Physicians (AAFP) holds the opinion that the "interests of patients are best served when their care is provided by a physician or through an integrated practice supervised directly by a physician." [145] Nurses, on the other hand, believe that collaboration, not supervision, is key. [145]

"We must learn to function as a true interdisciplinary team," says NP Jan Towers. [145]

While doctors may worry about the growing use of nurse practitioners; there's a clear consensus that they're needed. If only 2% of medical students are choosing to go into primary care, opting for higher-paying specialties, this need will only intensify. [149] A 2007 survey by the Commonwealth Fund found that only 30% of US citizens are able to get same-day appointments with a doctor when they are ill. [149]

Ted Epperly, president of AAFP says, "If we're going to be honest, the increase of nurse practitioners is a symptom of the disease. The disease is a lack of a robust, family, primary-practice physician network." [149]

Bernadette Melnyk, dean of Arizona State University's College of Nursing and Healthcare Innovation, says "People are so underserved in so many areas of our state. There is no need for territorialism here." [149]

What Doctors Say

Doctor Neil Brooks doesn't agree with the CAPNA approach; he emphasizes that doctors and nurses need to work in teams. "The end result of this extensive training and teamwork is truly comprehensive health care where patients are the winners," he says. [145]

Some doctors believe that NP-run clinics will end up driving up health care costs because without supervision, NPs will be more ready to admit patients to hospitals, order more tests or request additional consultations. [145]

Family physician Jonathan Harris says, "Worrying that we can be replaced by nurse practitioners says that we don't have a high image of what family practice is about, who we are and what we can do." [145]

Dr. Jeffry Hatcher says, "The economic reality is we can't spend more time with patients. Working with a nurse practitioner frees me to see the patients who need me most." [145] Hatcher says he couldn't do without his NP. He shares his patient load with Lowanna Wallace and he says that they review *each other's* lab test results and X-rays. [145] He doesn't supervise Wallace on every case but signs off on her charts. [145]

Dr. Harris says his practice uses NPs in a collaborative way: the NPs maintain their own patient panels. [145] He says it's been a huge success: "With very well-trained people, who understand what they can and can't do, there's tremendous synergy. Together, the physicians and nurse practitioners are much more effective than they are separately." [145]

Dr. Bruce Bagley says "Family physicians offer a different service to patients. With four years of medical school and three years of residency training, their depth of understanding of complex medical problems cannot be equaled by lesser-trained professional." [145]

Epperly says "The nurse practitioner replacing the family doctor is not good for America. To say a nurse practitioner can fill the shoes of a family physician, in terms of total comprehensiveness of care, is just not true." [149]

What People Say (And Studies)

Back in 1996, there were already a number of studies that showed "nurses provide excellent primary care," says RN Sue Whittaker. [145]

The American Association of Nurse Practitioners (AANP) found that so many people were choosing NPs because "they provide individualized care, focusing not only on health problems, but also on the effects health problems have on people and their families; they explain the details of health problems, medications and other topics to help people fully understand how to take care of themselves; and they ask about people's worries and concerns about their health and their health care." [145]

A 2001 study reviewed patient satisfaction with emergency nurse practitioners and that of doctor-nurse emergency teams. [147] The study found that:

- Patients were much more likely to receive health education and first aid advice from a nurse rather than from a doctor

- Written instructions, contact information and discharge advice were more often given by nurses than doctors

- People seen by nurses in emergency situations were much less worried about their health than people seen by doctor-nurse emergency teams

A 2002 review of studies took a look at whether upon first contact, NPs provided care equivalent to that of primary care doctors. [146] This analysis found that:

- Patients were more satisfied with NP care than that of doctors

- No differences in health status occurred

- NPs gave longer consultations than doctors did

- NPs made more investigations than doctors

- There was no difference in referrals, return consultations or prescriptions written

A 2006 overview of the work of physician assistants and nurse practitioners found that these professionals made up 1/6 of the medical workforce in the U.S. and these numbers are growing. [148]

The overview also found that the productivity of PAs and NPs matched that of physicians and that the range of services they provided compared to primary care doctors was 90%. [148]

NPs "have historically provided at least three times more health promotion and disease/injury prevention services than physicians or PAs," said the review and are the primary resource for an increasingly "out-stripped" medical force. [148]

Only 30% of US doctors practice primary care medicine while 50% of PAs and 85% of NPs do and they see 10% more patients yearly than do doctors.[148]

As far as fears about PAs and NPs increasing health care costs, the review found that per-patient health care costs were lower not only because of the lower salary of NPs and PAs but because they used less resources in terms of imaging, laboratory services, medication, referrals and garnered less return visits (probably due to the patient education they prescribe.) [148]

Roderick Hooker, author of the analysis, said that "Observers believe that traditional medicine can no longer sustain the old 'command and control' model of medical practice" and that physician, NP and PA practices are intersecting in a "shared domain" that is beneficial to U.S. health care. [148]

Qualifications and Regulations

NPs and PAs are regulated by individual state licensing boards. [148] Most states require that NPs work in collaboration with doctors but as of 2006, 16 states allowed them to practice independently and 11 of these states allowed them to write prescriptions independently. [148] PAs are usually required to work under the supervision of a doctor, with some form of communication. [148]

Roderick Hooker says that the scope of practice differs widely from state to state, defined widely in some and severely restricting PAs and NPs in others. [148] Hooker believes that this legislation "can sometimes provide a competitive edge for one profession over the other." [148]

NP Linda Pearson says, "As is often the case, we've worked to legitimize what nurse practitioners were already doing." [145]

Today, besides certification, NPs must hold a master's degree or higher. [145] They must complete 500 to 1,000 hours of supervised hands-on training and more accreditation programs are requiring a doctorate degree. [149] By 2015, it's expected that all NP programs will require a PhD. [149]

25 states and the District of Columbia now allow NPs to practice without physician supervision and mandatory collaboration. [149] All states allow NPs to write prescriptions and 17 of these don't require doctor approval of prescriptions. [149] Medicare now covers services provided by NPs and many HMOs now list them as independent providers. [149]

Pros and Cons

Dr. Jeffry Hatcher says, "It may make economic sense to bean counters to use nurse practitioners, but they don't have the training to function as *independent* practitioners. They're very good at handling single-system disorders, but when you get into multisystem disorders, you need a physician." [145]

Ted Epperly says, "I don't want to come across as slamming practitioners: my office has two. But to become a family physician, you need anywhere from 10,000 to 14,000 clinical hours." [149]

Dr. Tiffany Nelson says, "I think primary care is probably the hardest place for nurse practitioners to work because there is such a wide variety of problems and conditions we have to deal with. The common (problems) are easy to treat, but not everything is common." [149] Nelson believes NPs are better off in specialist's offices "where they are seeing the same thing over and over again." [149]

But nursing education focuses on primary care, preventive medicine and patient education, the stuff that benefits people in primary care the most. [145]

NPs focus on the communication and real care so increasingly cut out of the doctor-patient relationship today. NP Agnes Oblas says that with her own practice, she's able to offer a personal and one-on-one visit to her clients. [149]

"I only see maybe seven patients a day, which was unheard of where I was," she says. "There, it was sometimes 25 a day, in and out quick." [149]

She says that in today's health care system, too often "things fall through the cracks. People wait days or weeks for a referral. That's not going to happen to my patients." [149]

Dr. Jennifer Ashton still warns that as far as retail clinics in places like Walgreens and the like, "the buyer has to beware." [151] "The patient has to use the same amount of caution as if looking for a doctor," she says. [151]

Some clinics, Ashton says, offer very basic evaluations and treatments and are meant for minor ailments. [151] She thinks NP clinics are a good choice for travelers and otherwise healthy people but aren't a good option for those with chronic medical conditions or complicated health histories. [151] In some cases, she adds, the clinic may be operating with financial incentives to prescribe certain medications. [151]

In 2008, retail clinics in drugstore chains grew from 150 to 700. [152] The clinics are a draw because 90% of patients are walk-ins and the wait time is minimal compared to scheduling a doctor's appointment. [152]

One consumer remarked, "I got an appointment with my regular doctor last year for this same thing, and I ended up seeing a nurse practitioner there anyway. So I thought that I would go where I knew I could probably get the same experience in less time and with less hassle." [152]

Retail clinic visits are often short, about 15 minutes and there's rarely time to review a complete medical record. [152] You should clue in the NP about what medications you are taking and have them send a record of the procedures done to your family physician. [152] The clinics make use of electronic health records, which allow you to keep your PHR updated. [152] They're also more affordable if you don't have health insurance. [152]

Many retail clinics don't have room or time to perform X-ray machines and more complicated tests so conditions like fractures and mysterious ailments aren't what you want to try to have treated at these outlets. [152] They're also not a good choice for chronic pain prescriptions because many clinics limit those in order to combat drug abuse and addicted consumers. [152]

A 2006 survey found that those with no insurance or with very high deductibles were very pleased with the care that they received at a retail clinic and a 2007 Harris Poll found that 90% of retail clinic consumers were satisfied with their care. [152]

NP Nancy Dawson says, often "some people just want direction on what the next step in taking care of themselves would be." [152] That's where many retail clinics are really headed: preventive care and helping people to manage their own health. [152]

They're looking into downloading data from medical devices for patients with chronic conditions, and offering screenings such as those for cholesterol, diabetes, high blood pressure and skin cancer. [152]

Some of the clinics are even part of hospital systems and HMOs. [152] Some HMOs waive co-payments if a patient goes to a retail clinic but this might not always be advisable: sometimes a patient *should* go see their primary care doctor. [152]

The AAFP doesn't endorse retail clinics because it fears patients won't establish "medical homes:" treatment teams of primary physicians and other health professionals, relying on occasional visits to clinics instead and not following up with treatment. [152]

The most important consideration, when you come down to it, is that NPs are practicing the core principles of primary care, the principles family physicians have always espoused but are less and less likely (or able) to deliver: patient-centered care, the patient-doctor relationship, contextual healing that takes the family and community of the person into account. [145] They focus on patient education and empowerment and the prevention of disease.

A retail clinic is good for minor ailments, a more advanced NP clinic for more advanced conditions. If you have a complex condition or complex history; you're better off with a primary care physician. Your best bet is to establish a "medical home:" a network of professionals that includes physicians, specialists, nurse practitioners, pharmacists and the like all clued in to your unique health and working collaboratively.

Chapter 10:
Concierge Medicine

"Boutique medicine," "executive health programs," "platinum practices," "country club medicine," "retainer practices"...concierge medicine is called many things, including elitist. [154] It is also said that concierge medicine is worsening the doctor shortage going on in America today.

In 2004, there were only a small number of doctors choosing concierge service. [154] Today, it's estimated that there are more than 5,000 doctors practicing "direct care" and Thomas LaGelius of the Society for Innovative Medical Practice Design says "Patients love Marcus Welby health care. We are getting back to how medicine should be practiced." [155]

For an annual or monthly fee, a concierge doctor offers personalized medicine and the fee often covers procedures and preventive care that insurance companies wouldn't.

LaGrelius runs SkyPark Preffered Family Care and he charges from $950 to $1,900 for being available by phone 24/7 and making house calls. [155]

Darin Engelhardt of MDVIP says that the recession barely affected sign-up rates: the renewal rate in the MDVIP network in 2009 was 92%. [155]

Concierge doctors say that the rates of retainer fees average $4 to $5 a day, what most people spend on coffee and snacks. [155] "For that, you could get outstanding care," says LaGrelius. "What we are doing is mainstream and affordable. [155]

"In 2004, president of a boutique health care law firm Vasilios J. Kalogredis talked about the growing trend of concierge medicine. [154] He said that falling insurance reimbursements, paperwork and impossible patient loads triggered doctors to look for other options of practice. [154]

With retainer models, doctors end up with time to spend actually doctoring and patients end up with priority appointments, 24/7 cell phone and pager access to their doctor, house

calls, preventive, nutrition and wellness programs, telephone and e-mail consultations, free
check-ups and plenty of other perks. [154]

The History

Concierge medicine isn't really something new.
Dr. Michael Shahid crusaded to overthrow
fee-for-service practice back in 1900's. [156] He
founded the first cooperatively owned and managed hospital in Oklahoma. [156] He advocated
affordable, pre-paid health care by groups of
doctors and promoted the then-new idea of
preventive medicine. [156]

Shahid was motivated by the poverty of
farmers he saw and created one of the first
team models of pre-paid care. [157] In 1929, he
proposed that a number of doctors get together
and offer health care to farmers and their families for $50 a year that included all procedures
and treatments. [157]

At first, Oklahoma doctors tried to protect
their growing incomes and status by trying to
get Shahid's medical license revoked. [157] The
American Medical Association tried to suppress
cooperatives that were springing up around
the country because they "subjected doctor's
incomes and working conditions to direct control by their clients." [157]

President after president in America has tried to determine who should act as patient advocates and who should determine doctor's incomes. Government regulation is often tied to profit-minded groups like insurance companies and the pharmaceutical industry however. [157]

And even though it may seem at odds to have doctors have a hand at determining fees; people trust their doctor's decisions more readily than they do the government. [157]

Today

Dr. Shahid's model is how world-renowned Mayo Clinic and Cleveland Clinic run. [157] Medicare data has shown that these hospitals provide *less* expensive care with better health outcomes. [157]

Instead of the cookbook medicine that may result from current health care reform legislation, the team model and pre-paid idea gives doctors professional autonomy to prescribe the treatments they believe most effective instead of having to schedule tests and procedures insurers are willing to cover. [157]

Dr. Mark McClellan, former head of Medicare says, "It's a lot more accountability, which is why it's scary for physicians, but in some ways, it's also more autonomy." [157]

At a conference called "How Do They Do That?" in which practitioners and providers that repeatedly came under average cost growth gathered, McClellan asked how many of them thought fee-for-service was "archaic and fundamentally at odd" with good practice. [157] The majority raised their hands. [157]

Employers are among the people jumping on the concierge bandwagon. Chairman of the printing company Serigraph Inc. John Torinus, for example, has hired a doctor to provide free direct primary care to the company's employees. [158]

"If you keep people healthy, you're going to save health costs," Torinus says. [158]

Torinus had already built a Serigraph clinic that hosted a chiropractor, dietician, nurse coach and nurse practitioner. [158] He went through ModernMed Inc. to hire a doctor with a three-year contract. [158]

"I'm not paid on volume, I'm paid on satisfaction with care," the newly hired physician said. [158] He left his private practice to go with ModernMed Inc. who gets 30% of the fees. [158]

This doctor, like many others, is just fed up with not being able to manage patient loads, administrative tasks, the increasing number of salaries he must pay to handle the bureaucracy and the lack of real doctor-patient time.

Dr. Dragan Djordjevic is one of those doctors. [155] He used to see up to 30 patients a day for about 15 minutes each until a long-time patient of his called to tell him she was changing doctors. [155]

"She told me 'the last time that I saw you, even though it was for something relatively minor, it didn't appear that you were all there,'" remembers Djordjevic. "That left a bad taste in my mouth. She was right." [155]

The doctor decided he wanted less patients and more time with them and went "boutique" in 2007. [155] He limits his patient load to 600 patients, one-fifth of what he had to take on in order to keep afloat in his old practice. [155] He sees about 9 patients a day and meets with them for *at least* a half hour each. [155]

The $1,500 fee includes same-day appointments and 24/7 access to the doctor by cell phone or email. It doesn't include specialist fees or hospitalizations, which people still need health insurance for but Djordjevic says "Our system works wonderfully well. It focuses on prevention and wellness." [155]

Dr. Pauline Chen, who writes a doctor-patient column for *The New York Times* says that a Mayo Clinic survey has found that primary care residents spend as much as 6 hours a day in paperwork: spending as much time "writing, typing, or dictating about their patients as they do seeing them." [159]

Doctors have often complained that paperwork, including billing and insurance company blather, takes up most of their time. Insurance bureaucracy and paperwork account for *31% of every health care dollar spent in the U.S.* [161] The Physicians for a National Health Program say that streamlining the process could save more than $400 billion a year. [161]

Dr. Amy Oxentenko, who led the Mayo study said, "Resident's are learning a lot of medicine from the computer. That does nothing to foster the relationship with the patient." [160]

Errors due to fatigue are often attributed to the long hours medical residents are forced to endure but a new type of error is on the rise, says Oxentenko. [160] Residents are forced to make decisions about patient treatment with little time to get a comprehensive view because of paperwork.

"If you are spending so much time entering a note just because you have to enter a note, that's less time to review that patient's history, drug interactions, contraindications and the best test to order for that particular patient." [160]

Chen points out that EMRs can often become a substitute for doctor-patient interaction and doctors might end up relying on notes that are based on still other notes instead of making decisions based on any actual interaction with the patient. [160] This "cut and paste" process can often allow important information to get lost in the transfer, say Chen. [160] She likens it to the distortion of information that occurs with the childhood game "Telephone" or "Operator." [160]

The danger, says Oxentenko, is that as these habits become necessary for residents, they become lifetime practices for physicians. [160]

And it's not concierge doctors who are contributing to doctor shortages, say many. It's the fact that primary doctors are so overburdened and so under-compensated and the fact that medical students choose specialization and doctors leave the field after a few years. [155] Concierge medicine can offer comparable salaries and less administrative burden. [155]

Englehardt says, "We actually provide a vehicle that allows them to extend their careers." [155]

The focus on preventive medicine in concierge medicine, a practice that most primary care physicians have little time for today, means that "physicians can serve as a coach, not just as a treater of illnesses," says Englehardt. [155]

MDVIP patients are 40% less likely to end up in the hospital than people with normal health insurance and 74% less likely to be hospitalized than Medicare recipients. [155]

Changing coverage for concierge care might allow it to remain in reach for far more people and drive health care costs down.

"A lot of preventive stuff has fallen by the wayside," says Djordjevic. "If you don't have the time to listen to your patients, you are going to order an expensive test when a physical exam would have told you what you need to know. But if you can give patients the time, you can save the system money." [155]

Other doctors have similar views.

Juggling more than 3,000 patients and "getting squeezed by declining insurance reimbursements, Dr. Alan Sheff says, "I was going to leave medicine. Carpentry started to sound like a very good career option for me." [162]

Sheff shut down his practice and started charging a $1,500 annual fee for comprehensive care. [162]

Dr. Brent Cohen, found that seeing 25 patients a day and finding his practice "a blur of exams, office hours, referrals, hospital duties, reimbursement worries, staff management, forms and more" also considered a switch but after generating positive response from more than a third of his patients: decided not to switch. [163]

Why?

Even though he was tempted by the "long-forgotten luxury" of being able to spend time with patients, he was unsure of the future of the model. [163] He was unsure of whether or not insurance companies would contract with him, he was unsure about patient-discrimination laws, he decided in the end that he didn't want to abandon patients that might not be able to afford his fee. [163]

Michael Fleming of the AAFP says, "I have a great concern that this is going to provide care to the 'healthy wealthy,' but may limit access of the rest of the population." [163]

The ethics of making a move that will improve health care in the long run but leave people not covered during the shift has many doctors hesitating. [163]

They wrestle with the idea that if they switch; they'll limit access to health care for some of their patients until things change and yet funneling as many as 5,000 patients through a single doctor "often amounts to assembly-line medicine." [163]

Doctors like internist Benoit say "Even more so than I imagined, it's changed my life. I've gone from getting up in the morning knowing I can't possibly do everything I need to do...to being part of life. I can be more active in prevention. I always believed in prevention, but you had to deal with the matter at hand." [163]

He explains that of the 15-minute increments allotted to his patients in his former practice, 2-6 minutes were spent in the waiting room and 5-7 minutes were taken up by having weight and vital signs read. [163] That left 2-6 minutes with the doctor. [163]

"It's given me my profession back," Cohen says. "Instead of being reactionary, we have time to be proactive." [163]

Concierge medicine comes with other professional benefits as well. Dr. Robert Colton offers DNA profiles that analyze how individuals metabolize specific medications, a technology that would normally be inaccessible to most primary care doctors utilizing conventional insurance coverage. [163] Colton's practice requires a $2,100 initial fee for a profile and then a $250 annual fee to update it as patients take new medications. [163] Talk about personalized medicine!

Dr. Benoit says, "My family loves it. I have coffee with my wife in the morning. I play with the baby, and the older kids have time with me. I see them off to school, and sometimes I'm there when they come home. I feel very, very content." [163]

Cohen, on the other hand, thought "If you're going to be available 24/7, getting away is not an easy thing." [163] He heard from other doctors that had made the change that during the first 3-6 months, patients would call often "to make sure they were getting their money's worth." [163] Even though that lessened with time, Cohen worried that "you're still carrying that pager around all the time." [163]

Orthopaedic surgeon Dr. Peter Lavine said not only is the patient load and administration relief wonderful, the $1,500 retainer fee adds up to serious money, money that is lost to doctors in today's practice of medicine. [164]

Linda Nash was a former consumer who founded PartnerMD. [164] "A doctor's staff can be as dogged as gatekeepers," she explained. "It's all about keeping consumers away to maximize the physician's time." [164]

Partner MD negotiates rates with insurance companies and the annual fee doesn't cover deductibles and co-pays but offers quality to both doctors and patients. [164]

Sandra Ibrahim, an early recruit, says "I wanted continuity with the patient, to grow with them and become part of their family." [164] She didn't find it in conventional practice.

"It was urgent-care, pump-it-out, production-line work," she says. [164] "Yes, I'm a doctor," Ibrahim says, "but I'm also a mom, a wife, a sister and a daughter. I took a pay cut to come here—a $25,000 pay cut. That's how miserable I was." [164]

Now she sees a third of her former patient load and says, "You just get to know so much more about each person. I now have the kind of relationships with patients that took my former boss 15 to 20 years to make." [164]

Her work in preventive care is the real boon.

"Let's say a patient comes in for a physical, and his blood-glucose level comes back at 101. That's just barely prediabetic; normal is less than 100. In my old practice, we'd see how the patient did at his next physical. Or maybe we'd have him come back in six months. Here, when I get a level of 101, I have the time to research that. I'll go back and look at old records and try to pick things up in their family history, lifestyle, medications, or other factors. And I'll tell him: 'This is what I want you to do. I don't want to wait until you are diabetic.' That's pretty aggressive. In my old practice, we might have waited until the blood-glucose level was 120. But I don't want to wait. We're trying to catch those pink flags before they become red flags." [164]

That's the complaint many doctors have. Both Medicare and other insurance providers offer generous reimbursement to doctors for procedures but much less for office visits, gathering of history and conversation: key factors of health care. [164]

Dr Janice Ragland says that the reimbursement rate difference between specialists and primary care doctors illustrates that failing. "That gap used to be two to one. Now it's four to one." [164]

Family physicians, pediatricians and general practitioners are the lowest-paid doctors in US health care. [164] They make about $171,000 to $186,000 per year and you have got to consider their 12-year sacrifice to education and the hours they put in. [164] Specialists like radiologists and orthopaedic surgeons make from $400, 000 to $500,000 a year. [164]

Ragland says, "We spend probably 40% of our time on paperwork, phone calls, reviewing labs—work that doesn't get reimbursed." [164]

Dr. Sheff appreciates the quality standards MDVIP sets: staff has to answer the phone "by the second ring" and he gives patient written reports after their physicals. [164]

"I don't have to wear the business hat all day long. I'm back to being a doctor," he says. [164]

Doctors Mark Vasiliadis and Kevin Kelleher opened up their own concierge practice rather than going with a network. [164]

"We had the sense that we would be constrained in their practice model. Our goal was just to provide better and unique care: it wasn't to become concierge doctors." [164]

Even though many critics call concierge care elitist, Englehart of MDVIP points out that at $4 a day, it's a viable option for many. [164]

Some companies, like Privia Health, are combating the "country-club" view of concierge medicine. [164] They're building a doctor network in Washington that charges only $25 to $75 a month and employs preventive medicine practitioners like NPs and nutrition counselors. [164]

Cutting out the insurance company middle-man has its benefits. New Atlantic Ventures, for instance, invested heavily in Qliance, a company that offers "direct primary care" and for as low as $600 per year gives concierge benefits. [164]

Dr. Lori Heim of the AAFP says, "We all agree that you need to be really able to coordinate the care of your patient. If you do that, you'll have tremendous cost savings in the future. It's a whole lot cheaper for me to manage my diabetics than to pay for amputation or dialysis." [164]

Health reform today might eventually lead to retainer practice, where consumers would pay a monthly fee for a medical home model: a team of health practitioners that emphasize a holistic view of people's health care.

Medicare programs are looking into the possibility that the savings retainer-models generate could lead to cost savings for everyone after all. [164]

As far as doctor-shortages in the interim? Dr. Ibrahim says, "At the end of the day, I'm a happy practicing doctor, which I think is much more important than being a disgruntled doctor who's not practicing medicine." [164]

The website RangeIMD.com is run by a primary care doctor in Texas. [165] This doctor has quite a few very valid points to make in terms of comparisons concerning concierge and primary care as it is now. [165] This doctor clearly outlines and defeats the criticisms of concierge care: [165]

"Seeing fewer patients will reduce access to primary care."

This only applies to the assembly-line process that's in effect now. Many people only need a telephone or email conference to assuage their fears and others are well-served by NPs and PAs, says this doctor. Access is actually increased by concierge care and when doctors have more time to respond to patients; less referrals to specialists and unnecessary procedures occur.

"Physicians will have LESS incentive to see patients and perform care since they are paid up front."

This only makes sense for overworked and underpaid doctors, says Rangel. When they have real personal stake in the running of their practice, doctors are *more likely* to prove that their patients are well-cared for and have *more incentive* to incite their patients to renew their retainer fees. It's not going to middlemen!

"Only the 'rich' will be able to afford concierge care."

There are practices that charge country club prices, "many charge amounts that are comparable to the yearly cost of cable TV." And so many concierge doctors have the freedom to discount their fees according to economic capacity and medical need. That's not true with Medicare. Those rates are fixed and doctors are legally prohibited from charging less.

"Concierge patients get better care."

This factor is the biggest threat to the U.S. health care system. The actual numbers haven't yet come in that prove that concierge medicine results in better health outcomes but it only makes sense that this model will generate better health care. This is the basis for the "healthy wealthy" criticism.

"Concierge patients get better service."

Another threat to traditional health care and an issue of contention.

"Concierge physicians just want to get rich."

Yet concierge doctors greatly reduce the number of patients they see and take enormous financial risk in order to do so.

"Concierge medicine will increase health care costs."

In the long term, concierge care will reduce overall health care costs with its emphasis on comprehensive health care and preventive medicine.

"Concierge Medicine amounts to patient abandonment."

This is an issue many doctors wrestle with and is why they help their patients find other providers when they make the change. Technically, however, a doctor cannot be forced to work at financial loss or in a system that compromises patient care.

"Concierge Medicine is unethical."

The elitist argument says that this health care model is only available to those that can pay yet the present health care system doesn't cover 45 million Americans and the Medicare/ Medicaid system makes it illegal for doctors to treat patients at discounted rates.

In the end, concierge medicine is just one sign of a real health care revolution. It's re-empowering both doctors and patients and providing a holistic and team model for how health care should really work.

For people like Al Newland, who isn't wealthy, "The peace of mind for me is worth every penny." [164]

Chapter 11:
Medical Homes

Chronic health conditions place a massive burden on the health care system.

- 45% of the U.S. population has at least one chronic medical condition and many have several. [166]

- Among Medicare patients, 83% have at least one chronic condition and almost 25% have at least five. [166]

- From children to the elderly, 9 of 15 hospital admission diagnoses are the result of a chronic condition. [166]

- Chronic diseases cause 7 in 10 deaths every year in the US. [167]

- Nearly 1 in 2 adults live with at least one chronic illness. [167]

- The percentage of children with chronic health conditions have risen from 1.8% in the 1960's to over 7% in 2004. [167]

- The Centers for Disease Control and Prevention (CDC) says that 75% of US health care costs are due to chronic conditions. [167]

Chronic diseases, says the CDC, are the most common and most costly of all health problems but they are also the most preventable. Many of these conditions, from diabetes to heart disease, are related to four lifestyle habits: excessive alcohol use, poor eating habits, lack of physical activity and tobacco use. [167]

The current health care system doesn't provide tool and incentives to effectively manage chronic diseases: it rewards acute, episodic care, says Dr. Paul Keckley of the Deloitte Center for Health Solutions (DCHS), and doesn't cover proactive, preventive care. [166]

In 1967, the American Academy of Pediatrics (AAP) introduced a new health care model, the medical home, which is in the process of becoming a model for US health care. [168] A medical home, as described by the AAP in 2002, is "accessible, continuous, comprehensive, family-centered, coordinated, compassionate, and culturally-effective care." [168] This model may prove to be the nation's best bet in managing and preventing chronic conditions and better yet, it can help health care to move to a holistic, patient-centered, and team-based approach.

A medical home is not a physical place but a virtual home-base.

The American College of Physicians (ACP) defines a Patient-Centered Medical Home (PC-MH) as "a team model of care led by a personal physician who provides continuous and coordinated care throughout a patient's lifetime to maximize health outcomes." [169] This includes preventive medicine and coordinated care by a number of health professionals. It is made up of:

- A partnership between the family and the patient's health care professional

- Relationships based on mutual trust and respect

- Connections to services and supports for both medical and non-medical needs for the patient and family

- Respect for the family's cultural and religious beliefs

- After hours and weekend access to care

- Families who feel supported in caring for their family member

- Primary health care professionals coordinating care with a team of other providers

The American Academy of Family Physicians (AAFP), the American Academy of Pediatrics (AAP), the American College of Physicians (ACP) and the American Osteopathic Association (AOA) collaborated together to generate principles and standards for the PC-MH in 2007. [168]

The guiding principles for a PC-MH are:

- Each patient has an ongoing relationship with a personal physician who provides continuous and comprehensive care

- The personal physician is the leader of a team of professionals who work together to care for the patient

- The whole person is taken into account and care is for all stages of life

- Care is integrated across all elements of our complex health care system and community: hospitals, home health agencies, family, community-based services, and is facilitated by information exchange and technology so that patients get the care they need and want in "a culturally and linguistically appropriate manner"

- Evidence-based medicine helps guide decisions

- Doctors strive to improve the process with measures of performance

- Patients are active participants in decision-making

- Patients and families participate in quality improvement of the practice

- Access to care is enhanced

The National Committee for Quality Assurance is the accrediting agency for medical homes. [170]

Many doctors are embracing the medical home whole-heartedly. Patients with chronic conditions and complex diagnoses don't get coordinated care from the current fee-for-service system: it "rewards quantity of care over quality," experts say. [170]

Dr. Thomas Foels says, "The fee-for-service system is about driving up the volume of visits, and revenue depends on moving patients through the office. It is antithetical to the medical home." [170]

Dr. John Notaro says, "Everyone has been trained to work with patients one-on-one. Now, we're using a team, and we measure the out-comes, and we share those results among our-selves. That's a big change." [170]

Dr. David Pawlowski says, "I feel like the quarterback of a team." [170]

These doctors are using computers to identify at-risk patients, managing complex conditions with coaches made up of nurses, pharmacists and physician assistants to help people manage their own health, and they're using the latest scientific evidence for treatments and helping to measure their effectiveness. [170]

Buffalo Medical Group is one medical home model whose EMR was used to search through thousands of medical tests and records to iden-tify patients at risk for abdominal aortic aneu-rysms. [170] The electronic search identified 2,000 at-risk patients and further testing identified 30 people that were in imminent danger. [170] Anthony Antonik was one of those patients, with barely noticeable symptoms Antonik wouldn't have known "I was on the verge of death." [170]

There are still bugs to work out of the medi-cal home model, especially insurance and reim-bursement plans. Independent Health offers monthly care coordination payments to doctors and bonuses for reaching health outcome mile-stones like fewer hospitalizations. [170]

The changes in the way doctors are paid may prove to be difficult. A review of the model published in the *Annals of Family Medicine* said that the transformation of our health care system to a medical home model requires an "epic whole-practice re-imagination." [170]

It might take epic effort but recent reviews of the health outcomes are promising. The Patient-Centered Primary Care Collaborative (PCPCC) recently looked for the most credible studies. Here are six of those review results. [171]

1) Center for Evaluative Clinical Sciences at Dartmouth

U.S. states that rely on primary care have:

- Lower Medicare spending

- Lower Resource inputs (beds and labor)

- Lower Utilization rates (less doctor visits and hospital stays)

- Better quality of care

2) Barbara Starfield of John Hopkins University

- Adults with a primary care doctor are 19% less likely to die than those with specialist care and health care costs are 33% lower

- Primary care is linked with improved health outcomes for cancer, heart disease, infant mortality, life expectancy, low birth weight, self-care and stroke

- In both the UK and the U.S., every added primary care doctor per 10,000 people lowers death rates by 3 to 10%

3) Commonwealth Fund Report

- A medical home can reduce, and possibly eliminate racial and ethnic disparities in access and quality of health care

- Medical homes improve access, preventive medicine and management of chronic conditions

- Primary care of chronic diseases results in fewer complications and hospitalizations

4) RAND and the University of California at Berkeley

4,000 patients with asthma, congestive heart failure and diabetes were evaluated for the care they received according to PC-MH guidelines.

- Cardiovascular risk in diabetic patients was significantly lowered

- Congestive heart failure patients spent 35% fewer days in the hospital

- Asthma and diabetes patients were more likely to receive appropriate therapy

5) Mercer Analysis of North Carolina Community Care Operations

- The Medicaid pilot medical homes in North Carolina showed $244 million in savings for overall state health care costs in 2007

6) Commonwealth Fund Report on Denmark

- Denmark's entire heath care system is organized around medical homes and receives the highest patient satisfaction ratings in the world

- Denmark has the lowest per capita health expenditures and the highest primary care ratings

The Deloitte Center for Health Solutions also published a review of health outcomes with the use of medical homes and found: [166]

- The medical home model generated the greatest savings in heart disease and moderate savings in diabetes.

- Diabetic patients who participated in medical homes generated $137 less health care costs per month than patients who did not participate. The greatest savings came from a 22 to 30% reduction in hospitalizations.

- In terms of chronic heart failure patients, the cost of the medical home program was five times less than the savings in hospital costs.

- In an overview of 17 chronic conditions, there was a return of $2.90 for every dollar invested in the program, $41 in savings per member each month, 14% fewer hospital admission, 18% fewer emergency room visits, improvement in diabetic blood sugar levels and significant reduction in work and school absenteeism.

In March of 2010, researchers took a look at the medical home program in use at the Mattel Children's Hospital and the University of California. [172] The researchers found that after one year in the program, emergency room visits fell by 55%. [172]

Lead researcher Dr. Thomas Klitzner said, "The parents told us they felt empowered by the pediatric residents, supervising faculty and medical home staff to use scheduled outpatient primary care and specialty visits rather than using the emergency department to get care." [172]

Parents of children with complex or multiple medical issues often wrestle with managing the many appointments, medications, treatment plans and tests they're forced to deal with and socioeconomic barriers worsen health outcomes. The medical home helps parents to coordinate and manage their children's health. Bi-lingual liaisons, a binder that held all the medical records in one place and longer appointment times made a radical difference in the children's care.

Hopefully, the financial bugs will work themselves out and we'll all soon have the option of choosing a "home team" for our care. In the meantime, you might have to take on the quarterback role and lead your own team and coordinate your own care among the varied health professionals you see.

Chapter 12:
Complementary, Alternative and Integrative Medicine

Complementary and Alternative Medicine, Herbal Medicine, Traditional Medicine, Naturopathy, Holistic Medicine, Evidence-Based Medicine, Integrative Medicine

It's a bit bewildering today, the different terms used to describe different medical practices. Is traditional medicine the same thing as holistic medicine? Is naturopathy the same thing as herbal medicine? And what's integrative medicine?

The truth of the matter is that many of these terms overlap categories and as scientific research begins to prove the effectiveness of alternative therapies, it's likely that conventional medicine itself will require re-defining.

Complementary and Alternative Medicine (CAM) refers to any practice that isn't now considered a part of conventional medicine. Complementary medicines are those used to complement or supplement conventional medicine. Alternative medicines are those practices used *instead of* conventional medicine.

Herbal Medicine can be considered a CAM, a whole system or a component of other practices like traditional medicine or naturopathy.

Traditional Medicine is a complete medical system used in a specific culture and may include CAMs or be used as a part of holistic medicine.

Naturopathy is based on the belief that nature and all living organisms have a self-healing ability and the least invasive and most natural tools are used to restore balance and wellness.

Holistic Medicine is based on the idea that all things in nature and within our own lives operates interdependently. Holistic refers to the whole person approach in which health is made up of physical, mental, emotional and spiritual aspects.

Evidence-Based Medicine is supposed to be the cornerstone of conventional medicine, that is, it refers to practices that research has provided hard proof for in terms of effectiveness. The problem is, is that there is still a strong bias in conventional medicine to ignore evidence of efficacy in CAM and Traditional Medicines in favor of drugs.

Integrative Medicine is the newest addition to the practice of medicine. Many doctors are embracing the use of CAMs and other holistic therapies because science has found strong evidence for the mind-body connection to illness and evidence is beginning to mount for the effectiveness of certain herbs, acupuncture and other CAMs.

Integrative medicine involves using the best of all worlds to treat people holistically. It is a blend of conventional medicine and CAMs that have clinical evidence of efficacy behind them.

Complementary and Alternative Medicines (CAMs) [173]

You can investigate the evidence for a CAM therapy by visiting the National Center for Complementary and Alternative Medicines (NCCAM). They provide links to published studies and herb and supplement research as well as giving you guidelines to choose a CAM or a practitioner safely and wisely. Remember that "natural" doesn't mean "safe."

NCCAM divides CAM practices into four basic categories but many overlap. Whole medical systems cut across all four categories.

Whole Medical Systems

Whole medical systems are those that have evolved separately from and earlier than conventional medicine. They include Traditional Chinese Medicine (TCM) Ayurvedic Medicine, homeopathy and naturopathy. Many cultures and indigenous peoples still practice medicine distinctive to their cultures as their primary practice.

The World Health Organization (WHO) says that in some African and Asian countries, 80% of the population use traditional medicine as primary care and in developed nations 70 to 80% of the population has used aspects of traditional medicine as complementary or alternative therapy. [174]

Herbal treatments are the most popular form of traditional medicine and herbal supplements generated $5 billion in Western Europe from 2003 to 2004, $14 billion in China in 2005 and $160 million in Brazil in 2007. [174]

The four categories NCCAM divides CAMs into are Mind-Body Medicine, Biologically Based Practices, Manipulative and Body-Based Practices and Energy Medicine.

Mind-Body Medicine

Scientific evidence now supports the link between the mind and body in health. Cognitive behavioral therapy (CBT) for instance, was once considered a CAM but is now a conventional technique. Prayer, meditation, expressive arts therapy and other techniques that involve focus, posture and relaxation are still considered complementary or alternative.

Biologically Based Practices

Herbal medicine and substances found in nature used for healing are considered biologically based CAMs by the NCCAM.

Manipulative and Body-Based Practices

Chiropractic medicine and massage are examples of manipulative and body-based CAMs.

Energy Medicine

Energy medicine is based on the idea that the body operates and generates a force or field. Qi gong and yoga are thought to help balance the flow of energy in the body. Some energy medicine is based on the idea that electromagnetic fields exist within and outside the body. Magnet therapy and other electrical therapies fall into this category.

Ayurveda [175]

Ayurvedic medicine originated in India and is among the oldest medical systems. In Sanskrit, ayurveda means "the science of life." It is a holistic practice meant to balance and integrate body, mind and spirit. It involves universal interconnectedness, the body's constitution and life forces. Ayurveda employs many different CAM techniques from herbal medicine to yoga and has a strong focus on cleansing and harmony.

Traditional Chinese Medicine [176]

Traditional Chinese Medicine (TCM) is another ancient medical system and involves a wide variety of techniques including acupuncture, dietary therapy, herbs and qi gong. It is based on the principle that the human body is a microcosm of the universe and is interconnected to nature and its forces. Interdependence, balance, and the life force "chi "are important components of TCM.

Homeopathy [177]

Homeopathy originated in Germany in the 18th century. It is based on the principle that "like cures like," similar to the way vaccines work in the body. The idea is that diluted substances will stimulate the body's healing ability. Homeopathic remedies are produced from substances that are animal, mineral or plant.

Naturopathy [178, 179]

Naturopathy is a holistic European medical system that borrows from a variety of ancient and modern traditions and focuses on supporting the body's natural healing abilities rather than fighting disease. It is thought that a separation from nature suppresses healing and that the most natural and least invasive therapies are the best treatments. These include diet, herbal remedies, lifestyle changes and joint manipulation. Nature cures made up the first practices of naturopathy: the use of air, food, herbs, light and water. Lifestyle habits such as eating fiber and proper hygiene was a naturopathic contribution to conventional medicine.

The six principles of naturopathy are:

1) Promote the healing power of nature

2) First do no harm: minimize side effects and don't suppress symptoms

3) Treat the whole person

4) Treat the cause rather than the symptoms

5) Prevention is the best cure

6) The physician is the teacher and helps coach people to take responsibility for their own health

There are three kinds of naturopathic practitioners today: naturopathic doctors, naturopaths or other professionals that use naturopathic techniques. [180]

Naturopathic doctors have had four years of study in a naturopathic school; naturopaths may have learned through self-study or apprenticeship; chiropractors, doctors, nutritionists and other health professionals have a professional license but complement their work with naturopathic methods. [180]

Herbology, Herbal Medicine, Botanical Medicine, Phytotherapy

The use of herbs in medicine might be as old as the human race itself. Herbalism has been used before recorded history. [181] Although many people equate "natural" with "safe:" it's useful to remember that the field of pharmacology originated from the identification and study of plant compounds. The heart medication digoxin, for instance, is derived from foxglove and morphine comes from the poppy. [182]

Herbologists believe that whole herbs contain many known and unknown compounds that work synergistically in ways that isolated phytochemicals don't. [181] Herbal medicines involve use of both the whole plant and combinations of different herbs. [182]

A botanical is a plant or plant part that has medicinal properties: herbs are a subset of botanicals. [183] Botanicals come in many different forms, from teas and tinctures to extracts and decoctions. [183]

The environment a plant grows in, the harvesting and processing method and a number of other factors affects these compounds and how well an herbal medicine works. [181]

Dietary supplements aren't required to be standardized in the US and no definition for the standardization or consistency of a botanical supplement has ever been established. So, "standardized" on a label can mean any number of things and isn't a real measure of quality. [183]

In 2007, the FDA began requiring supplement manufacturers to meet Good Manufacturing Practices (GMPs). GMPs refer to identifying what compounds are in a supplement and identifying their purity and strength. [183] They're intended to help protect consumers from contaminants like pesticides and heavy metals and ensure potency but these are only guidelines. [184]

Manufacturers don't have to get FDA approval to put dietary supplements on the market even though they have drug-like actions. Producers of these products can make a variety of health claims as long as they also say that the FDA hasn't investigated or evaluated the claims. [184] The manufacturers are *supposed* to back up their claims with evidence but they're not required to submit this evidence to the FDA. [184]

The FDA takes complaints and reports of negative effects from supplement use and is supposed to then issue a warning or take action against the producer. [184]

It's best to do your own homework before using any kind of supplement and get advice from a professional.

The use of herbal supplements has greatly increased in the US but a study published in the *New England Journal of Medicine* found that 70% of people who do use herbs don't tell their doctor. [181] This can be very dangerous because herbs and other supplements can interact or interfere with other prescription medications.

A survey by the *Drug and Therapeutics Bulletin* found that most doctors believe that the public is not well-informed about herbal medicines but also found that 75% of the doctors themselves are poorly informed. [185]

Editor of the bulletin, Dr. Ike Iheanacho, said of the findings "It's obviously worrying that doctors in general seem to know so little about herbal medicines, given the widespread use of such products. The fact that few doctors make a point of asking patients whether they are taking herbal medicines raises further safety concerns. Similarly unsettling is that even when doctors don't know the effects of an herbal medicine a patient is taking, many won't try and look these up." [185]

You'll find many links in our resources section to do your own research on herbal and other dietary supplements.

Holistic Medicine

Holistic medicine describes any practice that takes the whole person into account: eating and lifestyle habits, stress and work, relationships and spirituality and all the factors that make up health and life.

In the 4th century, Socrates warned against treating just one part of the body "for the part can never be well unless the whole is well." [186] "Holism" was a term introduced in 1926 as a way of looking at all living things as "entities greater than and different from the sum of their parts." [186]

Conventional medicine focuses on symptoms and germs and isolated systems within the body. It focuses on curing or mitigating disease, uses drugs and surgery as its primary methods, and hasn't proved successful in the treatment of chronic conditions. [188]

Holistic medicine takes the stance that all things are interdependent and constantly interacting. [187] Lifestyle and mental attitudes are extremely important. It focuses on cures rather than symptoms, evaluates the whole person, and uses a wide variety of methods and patient empowerment to effectively treat both chronic conditions and acute diseases. [188] Holistic medicine is preventive and focuses on health instead of illness. [188]

The American Holistic Health Association says the holistic health means balancing and integrating physical, mental, emotional and spiritual components of your life, establishing cooperative and respectful relationships with others and the environment, making lifestyle choices that support wellness and taking active participation in your own health and healing. [187]

Integrative Medicine (IM)

Bruce Becker is someone who is grateful for the new practice of integrative medicine. [189] When an orthopedist told him he needed surgery for his tendonitis, surgery that may or may not work, he visited the Center for Pain Rehabilitation instead. [189]

Now, with acupuncture, electrical stimulus and physical therapy, Becker has gone from 15 to 20% use of his arm to 60% and he thinks he can get to 90%. [189]

Dr. Mitchell Prywes practices integrative medicine, the use of many different therapies to emphasize overall health, including body, mind and spirit. [189]

"We want to focus on health and wellness rather than disease system management," Prywes says and emphasizes that he still uses conventional medicine: "If I have pneumonia, I want antibiotics." [189]

Prywes prefers a low-tech approach and one with more doctor-patient interaction, more emphasis on patient involvement, and more diet and stress reduction techniques. [189]

Prywes teaches at the University of Connecticut School of Health, one of only eight medical centers in the US that has incorporated

integrative medicine into its family practice res-
idence program. [189] He teaches medical residents that a holistic approach that focuses on
disease prevention is more effective than using
the latest technology or the newest drug. [189]

Duke University has also embraced integrative medicine. [190] Duke has put out a pamphlet
that identifies the differences between conventional medicine and integrative medicine. [190]

Conventional Medicine	Integrative Medicine
• Manages disease	• Optimizes health
• Treats symptoms	• Treats the whole person
• Finds the problem and fixes it	• Identifies the risk and minimizes it
• Uses high-tech, bio-medical interventions	• Uses high-touch, whole person approaches
• Reacts to existing health issues	• Anticipates possible health issues and pro-motes prevention
• Intervenes as needed	• Plans across the lifespan
• Relies on the patient to achieve health goals	• Supports the patient to achieve health goals
• Directed by the physi-cian	• Guided by a partnership among patient, physi-cian and a team of clini-cal experts

Frederick Francisco is a doctor who has been
practicing integrative medicine for over a dec-

ade. [191] He explains that "We are saying there are other options—the natural, homeopathy, herbs, acupuncture. I look for what fits you, so I have to talk to you. I guide you on the options, but it's a two-way street—it's not just about me." [191]

Francisco stresses that both the mind and body need regular cleansing and detoxification. [191]

Dr. Andrew Weil is probably the most well-known practitioner of integrative medicine and is the founder and director of the University of Arizona's Program in Integrative Medicine. [192]

In a *Frontline* interview, Weil explains the purpose of the Consortium of Academic Health Centers for Integrative Medicine. [192] This purpose of the consortium, which consists of twelve prestigious schools and has many more waiting for inclusion, is to transform medical education. [192]

Weil says that medical students should be learning about nutrition, botanical medicine, the basis of mind-body medicine and how to survey alternative medical systems. [192]

Weil believes that medicine has to shift from focusing on symptoms and disease to healing and health. [192]

He stresses the idea that the body is built to diagnose itself, repair itself and regenerate itself and that his approach is to identify what's blocking those natural processes and help to facilitate the body's miraculous abilities. [192]

This revolution is well on its way and it's consumer-driven, claims Weil. He says that although conventional medicine holds that change should only occur after research, the reality is that people believe certain things and the research follows. [192] He points out that studies have found that doctors often don't change the way they do things in response to published research. [192]

There's still a lot of resistance to this movement, Dr. Weil says. He 's encountered three types. The first was resentment that these changes were being driven by consumers, the second was that many fear that the use of CAMs could be a slippery slope, and the third is simply peer censure and pressure. [192]

As far as the first, its high time medicine was directed by the patient rather than by doctors. The slippery slope theory doesn't hold water, says Weil, because the whole point of integrative medicine is discrimination, learning how to "separate the wheat from the chaff to find out what's worthwhile." [192]

As far as the third, as prestigious institutions and well-respected doctors come forth, this censure will loosen. He points out that after a talk he gave, when deans of medicine were asked to show their support for the teaching of integrative medicine; only one hand went up. But afterwards, in a written poll, 80% of those same deans said they were in favor of integrative medicine. [192]

Dr. David Eisenberg, director of OSHER Institute at Harvard Medical School, was also interviewed by *Frontline*. [192] He stresses that teaching integrative medicine doesn't mean that all doctors will be trained in acupuncture or herbal medicine, but that they can be trained to know enough to refer their patients to the proper specialists and successfully oversee their care. [192]

Eisenberg muses, "It would be wonderful, would it not, if in every part of the country, in every hospital, there was at least one doctor in every discipline—oncology, rheumatology, internal medicine and family medicine—who knew a lot about herbs, acupuncture and massage and could say, 'This is not safe, I wouldn't do that.'" [192]

"Wouldn't it be great," Eisenberg goes on to say, "if there were physicians who were expert in medicine as we know it, conventional biomedicine, who knew enough about complementary techniques and the approach to patient care to advise patients about the use or avoidance of individual therapies? And wouldn't it be great if their mindset was one of facilitating patient participation and encouraging the patient to do things that they could do for themselves? That's the future. I think that's what the public wants." [192]

So is integrative medicine for you? It might be your best fit if: [191]

1) You're open to new healing techniques and willing to give them time

2) You believe that you can heal yourself

3) You have faith in your doctor's capacity to help you heal

4) You are open and honest in your communication with your doctor

5) You have the ability to let go of unhealthy habits and mind-sets

6) You are open to building emotional and spiritual connection

Chapter 13:
HMOs, FFS, PPO and
POS Health Insurance Plans

As the U.S. health care system goes through its convoluted evolution, where are you left standing in terms of paying for health care? Managed health care is a system meant to control costs and delivery of health care. [194] The lofty goals managed care is *supposed* to aspire to include: [194]

- Helping health providers deliver high-quality care in a system that controls costs

- Ensuring that medically necessary care is given and that care specific to a patient's condition is given

- Making sure that the most appropriate health provider gives care

- Making health care available in the most appropriate and least restrictive setting

Managed health care plans have dominated in the US since the 1990's. These plans contract with doctors, hospitals and other health care providers to offer services to members at reduced costs. [193] HMOs and PPOs are the most popular health care plans but before the 1990's: FFS or Fee-For-Service was standard practice. [193]

HMOs

Health Maintenance Organizations (HMOs) are closed systems that are usually the least expensive and most fully reimbursed health care plans. [193]

For a monthly fee, you give up the freedom to choose your own doctors and can choose only from a list of providers that are members of the network. [193]

The primary care physician in an HMO is referred to as "the gatekeeper" and this doctor is the one who is supposed to manage a patient's care and refer them to specialists if needed. [194] If you see a specialist without such a referral, the HMO won't pay for it.

HMO's are the most restrictive insurance plan in terms of patient power and choice but they also offer a greater range of health services at the lowest prices. [194]

HMO Pros and Cons [195]

HMO Advantages	HMO Disadvantages
Low cost, low premiums, small deductible or no deductible, reduced co-payments	Doctor choice limited to providers included in the network
Minimal patient paperwork	You must have a referral to see a specialist
Coverage for some preventive care	There are limitations and qualifications for covered services
Choice from a wide range of services	

FFS

Fee-for-Service (FFS) plans are also known as indemnity plans. They are not managed care plans. [193] They are the most expensive health care plans but they offer patients the most flexibility and choice. [193]

In a FFS plan, you choose your own doctors and hospitals and encounter minimal interference when seeing a specialist of your own volition. [193] You pay quite a bit out-of-pocket and submit other bills for reimbursement. [193] Preventive services aren't usually covered and deductibles are high. [193]

Pros and Cons of FFS Plans [195]

FFS Advantages	FFS Disadvantages
Most patient choice	Costly in terms of money and time
You can change doctors at any time	You'll pay monthly premiums, a deductible and co-insurance costs
You can use any medical facility in the US	You have to keep receipts and fill out claim forms

POS

Point of Service (POS) plans are a type of plan offered by HMOs. They are also called HMO/PPO hybrids or "open-ended HMOs." [194] They're called "point of service" because the patient choose whether they want to used the HMO-style option or the PPO (preferred provider organization) each time they seek care. [194]

Referrals are made mostly by a primary care doctor but patients can see providers outside the network and still get some coverage. [193] If the primary physician refers out of the network of providers, the plan will pay all or most of the bill. [193] If you choose to see a provider not in the network; you'll have higher co-pays and deductibles and have to pay co-insurance fees. [194]

POS Pros and Cons [195]

POS Advantages	POS Disadvantages
You can see a doctor out of the network	You must still choose a network provider as a primary care physician who oversees your care
POS plans usually have more health and wellness and preventive programs than PPOs	You still need a referral from your primary physician to see a specialist

PPOs

Preferred Provider Organizations (PPOs) have more flexibility than the traditional HMO plan. [193] You don't have a gatekeeper but you'll get strong financial incentives to use providers within the network. [194]

You'll pay a set fee or co-payment for services and you can refer yourself to providers out of the network but you'll have to pay the difference in fees and pay higher deductibles and co-pays. [193]

PPO Pros and Cons [195]

PPO Advantages	PPO Disadvantages
There is a limit set on costs for network provider fees	Higher costs than traditional HMOs
You have unlimited choice in choosing a doctor if you're willing to pay more	More paperwork involved
You usually don't need a referral to see a specialist	Fewer preventive medicine services than traditional HMOs

Some other health care plans include COBRA and Health Savings Accounts (HSAs).

COBRA [195]

COBRA, the Combined Omnibus Budget Reconciliate Act of 1986, protects employees from losing their health benefits after losing their jobs. If you are fired, laid off or resign; your employer must continue your insurance coverage for a time. This doesn't apply to having been fired for "gross misconduct" and the time period is generally 18 months. This only applies to businesses that employ 20 or more employees.

If you lost your job between September 1, 2008 and January 1, 2010: the federal government will subsidize 65% of your COBRA premium payments.

Health Savings Accounts [196]

Some employers offer HSAs, Health Savings Accounts, which combine high-deductible health coverage with tax advantages. You pay high deductibles but lower monthly fees than you would in a PPO. The HSA then covers 100% of your care, unlike the 80% covered in a PPO plan.

This account is accruing, meaning that you don't "spend it down" every year: you build it up. Any money left over in your HSA account that you haven't spent on health services, is re-invested for the next year.

You choose your treatment. You can spend HSA funds on nutritional supplements, tests, CAM therapies or whatever treatment you choose.

An HSA provides you with tax savings by:

- Making your monthly contributions to the plan tax-deductible

- Your investment earnings in the plan are tax-free federally

- Making withdrawals for certain medical expenses is tax-free

Your annual deductible must be at least $1,150 for an individual and $2,300 for a family. The upper limits of your contributions to the HSA are $3,000 for an individual and $5,950 for a family. If you're older than 55; you can contribute $1,000 more a year.

If you enroll in Medicare, you can no longer contribute funds to an HSA but you can continue to use accumulated funds until the HSA is depleted.

There is a 10% penalty for using the funds for anything other than qualified medical expenses before age 65.

An HSA is a great choice if you're looking after your own health. It isn't so good if you continue unhealthy lifestyle habits and need constant and increasing after-the-fact care or prescription medications.

What to Look for in a Health Care Policy [196]

Charles Schwab offers some good guidelines for determining what coverage you should choose.

- Look for guaranteed renewable coverage, plans that can't be cancelled if you pay your premiums on time and don't hide conditions or otherwise defraud the company. This will protect you from the insurance company cancelling your coverage because you develop an illness.

- Look for a 10-day recission period. This gives you 10 days to really review the policy before you decide to keep it and still get a full refund if you decide otherwise.

- Read the fine print and get help to truly understand your policy, especially if you have a pre-existing condition.

- The Health Insurance Portability and Accountability Act of 1996 (HIPPA) is meant to protect you from exclusion because of a pre-existing condition. This only applies if you have had pretty much continuous coverage with no uncovered periods over 63 days.

- Catastrophic insurance is a high-deductible plan that offers a lower monthly premium for a higher deductible. This might be useful if you can't afford comprehensive care but want major expenses covered.

- If you don't have an established relationship with a doctor, an HMO might be a good choice.

- If you want more choice and flexibility, go with a PPO or POS.

- If you want to stay with doctors you're comfortable with, an FFS might be the only option.

- You should make sure you get additional coverage if your primary plan isn't adequate. The National Association of Health Underwriters (NAHU) and The Foundation of Health Coverage Education (FHCE) are good resources for finding independent insurance agents. You can find links to these organizations in our Resources section.

- Make sure your policy has a minimum of $1million in lifetime coverage. Serious injuries or illness can add up quickly.

Harvard University researchers found that *before* the most recent recession, in 2007, an American family filed for bankruptcy every 90 seconds after illness and 78% of them *were insured.* [197] Over 60% of all bankruptcies in the US in 2007 were due to medical causes. [197]

The researchers found that out-of-pocket costs averaged: [197]

- $17,943 for the medically insured bankrupt families

- $26,971 for the uninsured bankrupt

- $17,749 for those that with private insurance

- $14,633 for Medicaid patients

- $12,021 for Medicare patients

- $6,545 for patients with VA or military coverage

- $22,568 for families that started out with private coverage but lost it

Worse yet, most insurance coverage is linked to employment and 25% of US companies cancel coverage when a member suffers a disabling illness; 25% more cancel coverage within a year. [197]

Lead researcher Dr. David U. Himmelstein wrote: "The US health care financing system is broken, and not only for the poor and uninsured. Middle class families frequently collapse under the strain of a health care system that treats physical wounds, but often inflicts fiscal ones." [197]

Chapter 14: Conclusion

Current Status of US Health Care, Preventable Deaths: Lifestyle Choices, Emerging Models of Health Care, Power to the People

It's common knowledge that our health care system is in trouble, even in light of recent reforms. One president and one act are simply not enough to root out the insidious, pervasive and greed-over-good mentality that rules American health care.

It is up to us to take health care into our own hands, not only to live the healthiest lives we can; but to contribute to the changing of an unhealthy institution.

"Within each of us lies the power of our consent to health and sickness, to riches and

*poverty, to freedom and to slavery. It is we
who control these, and not another."*

~ *Richard Bach*

What are we really looking at in terms of the
status of health care?

Current Status of US Health Care

In 2000, WHO rated the US as 37th in health
care performance and 72nd in terms of the
overall health and quality of life for the average citizen. [198]

In 2006 the Commonwealth Fund compared
the health care systems of Australia, Canada,
Germany, New Zealand, the UK and the US in
regards to quality of care, safety of care, coordination and patient-centeredness, accessibility,
quality of life and expense. [199] The US ranked
last in every category except cost. [199]

Another study by the Commonwealth Fund,
published in 2008, evaluated 19 industrialized
nations in terms of their performance when
it comes to preventable deaths.   The result?
America came in last again. In fact, the study
found that in the years reviewed, had the U.S.
performed like the top 3 countries (France,
Japan and Australia,) 101,000 more Americans
would have lived. [200]

Preventable Deaths: Lifestyle Choices

Senate Finance Committee Chairman in 2009, Max Baucus, admits "Today, we spend nearly $800 billion on health problems that are directly linked to lifestyle and poor health habits each year—about one third of our total health care spending." [201]

Another report that the WHO puts out is about death due to chronic diseases. Cancer, diabetes, heart disease and chronic respiratory conditions are responsible for 60% of all deaths worldwide. [202]

Over 2.7 million deaths every year are due to low fruit and vegetable intake;

Over 1.9 million deaths are attributable to low physical activity. [203]

That's really a type of good news for the empowered patient: lifestyle changes can save 60% of American lives. Eating well, getting exercise, not smoking or drinking heavily can prevent you from developing a chronic disease.

If you can look at health care primarily as an individual responsibility and doctors and medicine as supplementary; you contribute to changing all American mentality.

If you can question everything; you'll find the kind of health care that suits you personally.

Your health is in your hands and there's plenty of help available to aid you in taking charge of it.

Emerging Models of Health Care

T. R. Reid, author of **The Healing of America: A Global Quest for Better, Cheaper, and Fairer Health Care**, says our best resource for determining what really works is the rest of the world. [204]

As far as the fear many have of socialized medicine, Reid points out that "almost all Americans sign up for government insurance (Medicare) at age 65," and "the US Department of Veteran Affairs is one of the planet's purest examples of government-run health care." [204]

As far as rationing, Reid says that German citizens can sign up for any of the country's 200 private plans and can switch among them with no premium increases; in France and Japan you must use a designated insurance provider but you can go to any doctor, any hospital and any traditional healer you want; and even though some countries do have waiting lists for non-emergency care; many of these countries outperform the US on waiting times for appointments and elective surgeries. [204]

Foreign health care systems are less bureaucratic and more efficient than the US. [204] In Japan, for instance, citizens see their doctors three times more than in the US, have twice as many MRI scans and X-rays but they spend $3,400 a year while the US citizen spends about $7,000. Plus, the Japanese have a greater life expectancy and better recovery from major diseases than Americans do. [204]

Some think that controlling costs will stifle innovation and yet some of the best research in the world comes from other countries. Deep-brain stimulation and hip and knee replacements were developed in foreign lands. In Japan, an MRI costs only $98 compared to the $1,500 they cost in the US yet the identical procedure still makes Japanese labs a profit. Cost control drove this innovation. [204]

Citizens with pre-existing conditions have to be accepted in other countries.

The key difference, Reid says, between health care systems in foreign countries and the US is that they exist to care for people's health. In the US, insurance companies are in it for profit. [204]

The US uses elements from many foreign health systems, says Reid. [204] For Native Americans and veterans, the care is British. For employer-based plans, we're like Germany. For those of us over 65, we're like Canada. [204] Reid says that this fragmentation is why our costs are so high: other countries choose one model and stick with it. [204]

Defenders of the American health system often say that the capitalist model has given us "the finest health care" in the world, says Reid, but the truth of the matter is we rank behind all other developed countries. [204]

Dr. Mary Jane England believes that until health becomes the focus of health care, until our system becomes patient-centered instead of profit-motivated, we're not going to get it right. [205] The financing must come afterwards, not first.

Preventive medicine, health coaches and Internet technology can help people to manage their own health. When health is the reward instead of providers being rewarded for visits and treatments, the system can really work and costs will fall. England says that the system must become one of "shared responsibility," that until every party becomes committed to doing their part to ensure the health of Americans; our system will remain a sick-care system. [205]

Power to the People

This book is meant to provide you with all the tools you need to take charge of your own health and help to change our health care system. The Internet is one of your most powerful tools. Yes, there are aspects that need fine-tuning and you have to be aware that the quality of information can differ widely among web-sites, but the Internet is probably one of the biggest factors driving the changes in American health care.

Susannah Fox of the Pew Internet Project has looked at the use of Internet health information among cancer patients. [206]

She found that Internet use was associated with better patient-provider relationships, better question-asking and better compliance with treatment. [206] Internet use was also associated with higher rates of self-efficacy, the confidence that patients had to make decisions and influence their outcomes. [206]

Fox has conducted quite a bit of research concerning the Internet and health care in America and she's found that the Internet is the means not the end, which can "accelerate the pace of discovery, widen social networks, and sharpen the questions someone might ask." [207]

One of the biggest benefits of the Internet is the social support people with chronic conditions or diseases encounter. Homebound people can build social networks. John Linna, who had to stay home on a ventilator and began a blog said: "That day my little world began to expand. Soon I had a little neighborhood. It was like stopping in for coffee every day just to see how things were going." [208]

Susan Fultz has found it helpful to commiserate with others that have mysterious ailments and trouble getting diagnoses. She has Lyme disease and psoriatic arthritis. "There's no worry of being judged or criticized, and that is something that I know a lot of us don't get in our daily lives." [208]

These networks also provide the everyday information and advice that many people need to determine how to best live with their disease.

One diabetic says, "I don't like to talk to my family and friends about this. I just really need some advice and people to talk to who might have been experiencing the same things." [208]

Another says, "There's no doctor in the world, unless they've actually lived with this thing, that can get into that nitty-gritty." [208]

Lily Vadakin, diagnosed with multiple sclerosis, says she's talked with others about what works to combat fatigue. "That's what the community can give you—a real-life perspective." [208]

Fox advises doctors, businesses, government and other agencies to take note of patient networks. [209] She says that they spread ideas, approaches and treatment information and that they can help providers innovate in patient-centered ways. [209]

In her article, "The Patient is In," Fox says, "Patients and the people who love them are not just your target audience, but your colleagues. They are a resource for innovation and knowledge." [209]

The Internet, says Fox, has given rise to "participatory medicine."

The empowered patient, the informed health consumer, is driving the evolution of the American health care system. Taking control of your own health care has been proven to produce better health outcomes and healthier people are better equipped to contribute to the real revolution of our nation's system.

"He who has health has hope; and he who has hope has everything."

~Arabic Proverb

Resources

Advertising

- **Federal Trade Commission (FTC)**

  http://www.ftc.gov/

- **Dietary Supplements: An Advertising Guide for Industry**

  http://www.ftc.gov/bcp/edu/pubs/business/adv/bus09.shtm

- **"Miracle" Health Claims: Add a Dose of Skepticism**

  http://www.ftc.gov/bcp/edu/pubs/consumer/health/hea07.shtm

CAMs

➢ **National Center of Complementary and Alternative Medicine**

http://nccam.nih.gov/health/clearing-house/

Doctors

➢ **AMA Doctor Finder**

http://www.ama-assn.org/aps/amahg.htm

➢ **The "Handoff": Your Roadmap to a New Doctor's Care**

http://www.cfah.org/hbns/preparedpa-tient/Prepared-Patient-Vol1-Issue4.cfm

➢ **Giving Your Doctor the Pink Slip**

http://www.cfah.org/hbns/preparedpa-tient/Prepared-Patient-Vol1-Issue8.cfm

➢ **Sorting Out Medical Opinion Overload**

http://www.cfah.org/hbns/preparedpa-tient/Vol2/Prepared-Patient-Vol2-Issue2.cfm

Drugs

> **MedScape**
> http://www.medscape.com/

> **Buying Medicines and Medical Products Online**
> http://www.fda.gov/buyonline/

> **Buying Prescription Medicine Online: A Consumer Safety Guide**
> http://www.fda.gov/buyonlineguide/

> **Beware of Online Cancer Fraud**
> http://www.fda.gov/consumer/updates/cancerfraud061708.html

> **Coping With the High Costs of Prescriptions**
> http://www.cfah.org/hbns/preparedpatient/Vol2/Prepared-Patient-Vol2-Issue3.cfm

Health Information

> **Medline Plus**
> http://medlineplus.gov/

> **Nutrition.gov**
> http://www.nutrition.gov/nal_display/index.php?info_center=11&tax_level=1

> **eMedicine Health**
> http://www.emedicinehealth.com/

> **Genetics Home Reference**
> http://ghr.nlm.nih.gov/

> **Household Products Database**
> http://hpd.nlm.nih.gov/

Insurance

> **COBRA**
> http://www.dol.gov/ebsa/faqs/faq_consumer_cobra.html

> **HSAs**
> http://www.ustreas.gov/offices/public-affairs/hsa/

Internet

> **Medical Products and the Internet: A Guide to Finding Reliable Information**

http://apps.who.int/medicinedocs/en/d/
Js2277e/

➢ **Navigating for Health: Finding Accurate Information on the Internet**

http://www.foodinsight.org/

➢ **US Health and Human Services: Quality of Health Information**

http://www.healthfinder.gov/scripts/
SearchContext.asp?topic=14310&section=5

➢ **10 Things to Know About Evaluating Medical Resources on the Web**

http://nccam.nih.gov/health/webre
sources/

➢ **CAPHIS 2010 Top 100 List: Websites You Can Trust**

http://caphis.mlanet.org/consumer/
top100all.pdf

➢ **Health on The Net Foundation**

http://www.hon.ch/

➢ **Medhunt**

http://www.hon.ch/HONsearch/Patients/
medhunt.html

PHR Accreditation

> **EHNAC**
> http://www.ehnac.org/accredited-organi-zations.html

> **CCHIT**
> http://www.cchit.org/products

> **CORE**
> http://www.caqh.org/search.php?query=cdc

> **HRCI**
> http://www.hrci.org/Page.aspx?id=2147483887

Privacy

> **Your Health Information Privacy Rights**
> http://www.hhs.gov/ocr/privacy/hipaa/understanding/consumers/consumer rights.pdf

> **Notice of Privacy Practices for the Original Medicare Plan**
> http://www.medicare.gov/privacyprac-tices.asp

> ➢ **How to File a Health Information Privacy Complaint with the Office for Civil Rights**
>
> http://www.hhs.gov/ocr/civilrights/complaints/index.html

> ➢ **HIPPA**
>
> http://www.hipaa.org/

Research

> ➢ **How to Understand and Interpret Food and Health-Related Scientific Studies**
>
> http://www.foodinsight.org/

> ➢ **10 Things to Know About Evaluating Medical Resources on the Web**
>
> http://nccam.nih.gov/health/webresources/

> ➢ **How to Understand and Interpret Food and Health-Related Scientific Studies**
>
> http://www.foodinsight.org/

> ➢ **Making Sense of Health and Nutrition News**
>
> http://www.foodinsight.org/

➢ **Deciphering Medspeak**
http://www.mlanet.org/resources/med-speak/index.html

Studies

➢ **BioMed Central**
http://www.biomedcentral.com/home/

➢ **PubMed**
http://www.ncbi.nlm.nih.gov/sites/entrez

➢ **International Bibliographic Information on Dietary Supplements**
http://ods.od.nih.gov/Health_Information/IBIDS.aspx

➢ **Public Library of Science**
http://www.plos.org/

Ongoing Research: Open Clinical Trials

➢ http://www.centerwatch.com/

➢ http://clinicaltrials.gov

Supplements

➢ Office of Dietary Supplements
http://ods.od.nih.gov/

➢ US Food and Drug Administration (FDA)
http://www.fda.gov/

➢ Claims That Can be Made for Conventional Foods and Dietary Supplements
http://www.fda.gov/Food/LabelingNutrition/LabelClaims/ucm111447.htm

➢ FDA Dietary Supplement Overview
http://www.fda.gov/Food/DietarySupplements/ConsumerInformation/ucm110417.htm

➢ Vitamin and Mineral Supplements
http://www.nlm.nih.gov/medlineplus/vitamins.html

➢ Tips for the Savvy Supplement User: Making Informed Decisions and Evaluating Information
http://www.fda.gov/Food/DietarySupplements/ConsumerInformation/ucm110567.htm

Watch Dog Sites

> **Non Profit Organizations with Ties to Industry**
> http://www.cspinet.org/integrity/corp_funding.html

> **MedWatch**
> http://www.fda.gov/Safety/MedWatch/default.htm

> **Quackwatch**
> http://www.quackwatch.com/

> **Sourcewatch**
> http://www.sourcewatch.org/index.php?title=SourceWatch

> **Center for Science in the Public Interest**
> http://www.cspinet.org/

> **CenterWatch**
> http://www.centerwatch.com/

Other/General and Comprehensive

> **Allies in Healthcare**
> http://www.alliesinhealth.com/home.asp

➢ **Center for Advancing Health**
http://www.cfah.org/index.cfm

➢ **AHIMA**
http://www.ahima.org/

➢ **Decision Tree**
http://thedecisiontree.com/blog/thomas-goetz/

References

1) Frontline Interview (2003, Nov. 4). Pros and Cons of Integrative Medicine. *PBS* [online]. Retrieved from http://www.pbs.org/wgbh/pages/frontline/shows/altmed/clash/integrated.html

2) Pew Internet (2005). Health Information Online: Summary of Findings. *Pew Internet & American Life Project* [online]. Retrieved from http://www.pewinternet.org/Reports/2005/Health-Information-Online.aspx?r=1

3) Goetz, Thomas (2010). **The Decision Tree: Taking Care of Your Health in the New Era of Personalized Medicine.** *Rodale Press* [online]. Retrieved from http://www.thedecisiontree.com/blog/

4) Goetz, Thomas (2009, Dec. 22). Welcome to the Era of Personalized Medicine.

The Huffington Post [online]. Retrieved from http://www.huffingtonpost.com/thomas-goetz/welcome-to-the-era-of-per_b_399911.html

5) Shah, Anup (2009, Nov. 4). Pharmaceutical Corporations and Medical Research. *Global Issues* [online]. Retrieved from http://www.globalissues.org/article/52/pharmaceutical-corporations-and-medical-research

6) Bass, Alison (2008, May 11). How Drug Advertising Misleads Consumers. *Alison Blass Blogspot* [online]. Retrieved from http://alison-bass.blogspot.com/2008/05/ever-wonder-why-there-are-so-many-drug.html

7) Shankar P R, Subish P (2007). Disease Mongering. *Singapore Medical Journal* [online]. Retrieved from http://www.encognitive.com/files/Pharmaceutical%20Industry%20Disease%20Mongering.pdf

8) Cassels, Alan and Moynihan, Ray (2006). US: Selling To the Worried Well. *Le Monde diplomatique* [online]. Retrieved from http://mond-ediplo.com/2006/05/16bigpharma

9) Heath, Iona (2005, Apr. 23). Who needs health care—the well or the sick? *British Medical Journal* [online]. Retrieved from http://www.ncbi.nlm.nih.gov/pmc/articles/PMC556345/

10) Null, Gary PhD; Dean, Carolyn MD, ND; Feldman, Martin MD; Rasio, Debora MD; Smith, Dorothy PhD (2006, August). Death by Medicine. *Life Extension Magazine* [online]. Retrieved from http://www.lef.org/magazine/mag2006/aug2006_report_death_01.htm

11) PR Log (2008, Oct. 1). Global Pharmaceutical Market Forecast to 2012. *PR Log Press Release* [online]. Retrieved from http://www.prlog.org/10124036-global-pharmaceutical-market-forecast-to-2012.html

12) PR Inside (2009, Jun. 2). US Pharmaceutical Industry Report, 2008-2009. *PR Inside* [online]. Retrieved from http://www.pr-inside.com/us-pharmaceutical-industry-report-r1291427.htm

13) Taragana (2010, Mar. 10). Pharmaceutical industry group spent $6.3M lobbying in Q4, on health overhaul, other issues. *Taragana Business News* [online]. Retrieved from http://blog.taragana.com/business/2010/03/10/pharmaceutical-industry-group-spent-63m-lobbying-in-q4-on-health-overhaul-other-issues-40041/

14) Ismail, M. Asif (2008, Jun. 24). A Record Year for the Pharmaceutical Lobby in '07. *The Center for Public Integrity* [online]. Retrieved from http://projects.publicintegrity.org/rx/report.aspx?aid=985

15) GovTrack (2008). Public Research in the Public Interest Act of 2006. *GovTrack* [online]. Retrieved from http://www.govtrack.us/congress/bill.xpd?bill=s109-4040

16) Sourcewatch (2009, Dec. 29). Pharmaceutical Research and Manufacturers of America. *Source Watch* [online]. Retrieved from http://www.sourcewatch.org/index.php?title=Pharmaceutical Research and Manufacturers of America

17) Enig, Mary PhD and Fallon, Sally (2000, February). The Skinny on Fats. *The Weston A. Price Foundation* [online]. Retrieved from http://www.westonaprice.org/The-Skinny-on-Fats.html

18) Weston A. Price Brochure (1999). Principles of Healthy Diets. *The Weston A. Price Foundation* [online]. Retrieved from http://trit.us/brochures/wapfbrochure.html

19) Sardi, Bill (2008, Jan. 21). Government Health Agencies Complicit in Cholesterol Ruse. *Lew Rockwell* [online]. Retrieved from http://www.lewrockwell.com/sardi/sardi79.html

20) Enig, Mary PhD and Fallon, Sally (2004, Jun. 14). Dangers of Statin Drugs: What You Haven't Been Told About Popular Cholesterol-Lowering Medicines. *The Weston A. Price Foundation* [online]. Retrieved from http://www.westonaprice.org/Dangers-of-Statin-Drugs-What-You-

Havent-Been-Told-About-Popular-Cholesterol-Lowering-Medicines.html

21) Eggen, Dan and Stein, Rob (2009, Nov. 18). Mammograms and politics: Task force stirs up a tempest. *The Washington Post* [online]. Retrieved from http://www.washingtonpost. com/wpdyn/content/article/2009/11/17/ AR2009111704197.html

22) Daily Mail (2006, Jun. 27). Mammograms 'Can Increase Breast Cancer Risk'. *Daily Mail* [online]. Retrieved from http://www.dailymail. co.uk/health/article-392619/Mammograms-increase-breast-cancer-risk.html

23) Press Release (2009, Dec. 1). Mammography may increase breast cancer risk in some high-risk women. *Radiological Society of North America* [online]. Retrieved from http://www. eurekalert.org/pub_releases/2009-12/rson-mmi112409.php

24) White, Edward MD and Stöppler, Melissa Conrad (2008, Feb. 26). Breast Cancer Prevention. *Medicine Net* [online]. Retrieved from http://www.medicinenet.com/breast_cancer_ prevention/article.htm

25) Nunes, Anthony (2010). Mammograms May Increase Risk Of Cancer. Consider Thermography As An Alternative. *Healthy for Life at Anthony Nunes* [online].

Retrieved from http://www.anthonynunes.com/ monthly article/mammograms.html

26) PBS (2003, Nov. 1). Dangerous Prescriptions. *PBS Frontline* [online]. Retrieved from http://www.pbs.org/previews/frontline_dangerous_prescription/PBS (2008). P

27) Chicago Tribune (2008, Oct. 23). Almost half of U.S. doctors use placebos. *The Chicago Tribune* [online]. Retrieved from http:// newsblogs.chicagotribune.com/triage/2008/10/ almost-half-of.html#more

28) Chicago Tribune (2008, Oct. 26). Placebos and the doctor-patient relationship. *The Chicago Tribune* [online]. Retrieved from http:// newsblogs.chicagotribune.com/triage/2008/10/ placebos-and-th.html#more

29) Niemi, Maj-Britt (2009, February). Placebo Effect: A Cure in the Mind. *The Scientific American* [online]. Retrieved from http://www. innerharmonyhypnosis.com/hypnosis articles/ placebo effect a cure in the mind scientific american.htm

30) Devlin, Hannah (2009, Oct. 16). Placebo effect starts in the spine – not just the mind. *The Times* [online]. Retrieved from http://www. timesonline.co.uk/tol/news/science/medicine/ article6877064.ece

31) Sidoti, Liz (2010, Apr. 18). Poll: 4 out of 5 Americans don't trust Washington. *The Associated Press* [online]. Retrieved from http://www.14wfie.com/Global/story.asp? S=12332069

32) Gruman, Jessie (2009, Feb. 25). Cost of Healthcare Transparency Is Trust in the American System. *US News* [online]. Retrieved from http://www.usnews.com/articles/opinion/2009/02/25/cost-of-healthcare-transparency-is-trust-in-the-american-system.html

33) SEED (2010). History of Medicine. *Schlumberger Excellence in Educational Development* [online]. Retrieved from http://www.seed.slb.com/content.aspx?id=30290

34) Goetz, Thomas (2010, Jan. 14). 3 Ways to Take Control of Your Health Today. *The Huffington Post* [online]. Retrieved from http://www.huffingtonpost.com/thomas-goetz/3-ways-to-take-control-of_b_417460.html

35) Stewart M; Brown JB; Donner A; McWhinney IR; Oates J; Weston WW and Jordan J (2000, September). The Impact of Patient-Centered Care on Outcomes. *The Journal of Family Practice* [online]. Retrieved from http://www.ncbi.nlm.nih.gov/pubmed/11032203

36) Press Release (2010, Feb. 24). Surgeon General with Microsoft Healthvault Expands

Consumer Benefits for the My Family Health Portrait Offering. *Office of Public Health and Science* [online]. Retrieved from http://www.hhs.gov/news/press/2010pres/02/20100224a.html

37) ACRL (2010). ACRL Legislative Agenda 2010: Public Access to Federally Funded Research. *Association of College and Research Libraries* [online]. Retrieved from http://www.ala.org/ala/mgrps/divs/acrl/issues/washingtonwatch/10agenda.cfm

38) NIH (2005, June). The End of One-Size-Fits-All Medicine? *The National Institutes of Health* [online]. Retrieved from http://newsinhealth.nih.gov/2005/June2005/docs/01features_01.htm

39) Durgin, Jennifer (2006). Pharmacogenomics: One size doesn't fit all. *Dartmouth University* [online]. Retrieved from http://dartmed.dartmouth.edu/winter06/html/vs_pharmacogenomics.php

40) My Personal Health Record (2010). What is Healthcare Literacy? *AHIMA Foundation* [online]. Retrieved from http://www.myphr.com/index.php/health_literacy/what_is_health_literacy/

41) My PHR (2010, Apr. 6). Health Literacy Cuts Costs, Increases Well-Being. *AHIMA* [online].

Retrieved from http://www.myphr.com/index. php/blogs/seniors/article/2348/

42) Goetz, Thomas (2010, Feb. 16). How to Make Better Decisions for Your Health. *The Huffington Post* [online]. Retrieved from http:// www.huffingtonpost.com/thomas-goetz/how-to-make-better-decisi_b_462830.html

43) Health Behavior News Service (2007, September). Effective Patienthood Begins With Good Communication. *Health Behavior News Service* [online]. Retrieved from http://www. cfah.org/hbns/preparedpatient/Prepared-Patient-Vol1-Issue3.cfm

44) Dartmouth Institute (2010). Inside the Drug Facts Box. *Dartmouth Institute* [online]. Retrieved from http://dartmed.dartmouth.edu/ spring08/html/disc_drugs_we.php

45) Wiencke, Matthew C. Patients deserve data about drugs. *Dartmouth Institute* [online]. Retrieved from http://dartmed.dartmouth.edu/ spring08/html/disc_drugs.php

46) Darmouth University (2008). Lunesta Box. *Dartmouth University* [online]. Retrieved from http://dartmed.dartmouth.edu/spring08/pdf/ disc_drugs_we/lunesta_box.pdf

47) MLA (2010). Deciphering Medspeak. *Medical Library Association* [online]. Retrieved from-

http://www.mlanet.org/resources/medspeak/index.html

48) Thorton, Amanda (2010). Authors aim to bring clarity to health statistics. *Dartmouth Institute* [online]. Retrieved from http://dartmed.dartmouth.edu/winter07/html/vs_authors.php

49) NIA (2003, 2006). Understanding Risk: What Do Those Headlines Really Mean? *National Institute of Aging* [online]. Retrieved from http://www.nia.nih.gov/HealthInformation/Publications/risk.htm

50) HSL and UNC (2004). **Introduction to Evidence-Based Medicine 4**[th] **edition:** "Types of Questions and Studies". *Duke University Medical Center Library and UNC-Chapel Hill Health Sciences Library* [online]. Retrieved from http://www.hsl.unc.edu/services/tutorials/ebm/supplements/questionsupplement.htm

51) The National Commission for the Protection of Human Subjects of Biomedical and Behavioral Research (1979, Apr. 18). The Belmont Report: Ethical Principles and Guidelines for the Protection of Human Subjects of Research. *National Institutes of Health* [online]. Retrieved from http://ohsr.od.nih.gov/guidelines/belmont.html

53) Pew Internet (2005). Health Information Online: Summary of Findings. *Pew Internet &*

American Life Project [online]. Retrieved from http://www.pewinternet.org/Reports/2005/Health-Information-Online.aspx?r=1

54) Markoff, John (November 24, 2008): "Microsoft Examines Causes of 'Cyberchondria';" *The New York Times* [online]. Retrieved from http://www.nytimes.com/2008/11/25/technology/internet/25symptoms.html

55) White R and Hovitz E(November 2008): "Cyberchondria: Studies of the Escalation of Medical Concerns in Web Search;" *Microsoft Research* [online]. Retrieved from http://research.microsoft.com/apps/pubs/default.aspx?id=76529

56) Usborne, Simon (February 17, 2009): "Cyberchondria: The perils of internet self-diagnosis;" *The Independent* [online]. Retrieved from http://www.independent.co.uk/life-style/health-and-families/features/cyberchondria-the-perils-of-internet-selfdiagnosis-1623649.html

58) Seligman, Katherine (2004, Feb. 15). Imaginary maladies online / Internet spreads 'cyberchondria'. *The Chronicle* [online]. Retrieved from http://articles.sfgate.com/2004-02-15/living/17410960_1_health-fears-health-information-pew-internet

59) Vardigan, Benji (2009, May 28). Fear of illness is the illness itself, and health information on the Internet is fueling the phobia. *Caremark* [online]. Retrieved from https:// www.caremark.com/wps/portal/HEALTH RESOURCES?topic=hypochondria

60) Ishikawa H; Yano E; Fujimori S; Kinoshita M; Yamanouchi T; Yoshikawa M; Yamazaki Y and Teramoto T (2009, Dec. 26). Patient health literacy and patient-physician information exchange during a visit. *The Journal of Family Practice* [online]. Retrieved from http://www. ncbi.nlm.nih.gov/pubmed/19812242

61) Sandberg EH and Sandberg PD (2009). A controlled study of the effects of patient information-elicitation style on clinician information-giving. *Community Medicine* [online]. Retrieved from http://www.ncbi.nlm.nih.gov/ pubmed/19798837

62) Hungerford, DS (2009, September). Internet access produces misinformed patients: managing the confusion. *Orthopedics* [online]. Retrieved from http://www.ncbi.nlm.nih.gov/ pubmed/19751023

63) Kim J and Kim S (2009, September). Physicians' perception of the effects of Internet health information on the doctor-patient relationship. *Informatics for Health and Social Care*

[online]. Retrieved from http://www.ncbi.nlm.
nih.gov/pubmed/19670004

64) Corcoran TB; Haigh F; Seabrook A and Schug SA (2009, September). The quality of internet-sourced information for patients with chronic pain is poor. *The Clinical Journal of Pain* [online]. Retrieved from http://www.ncbi.nlm.nih.gov/pubmed/19692804

65) News Staff (2010, Apr. 12). Internet health advice 'very variable', say city experts. *This is Nottingham* [online]. Retrieved from http://www.thisisnottingham.co.uk/news/Internet-health-advice-variable-say-city-experts/article-2001314-detail/article.html

66) Purcell, Gretchen P, Wilson, Petra and Delamothe, Tony (2002, Mar. 9). The Quality of Health Information on the Internet. *British Medical Journal* [online]. Retrieved from http://www.bmj.com/cgi/content/extract/324/7337/557

67) Hartzband, Pamela MD and Groopman, Jerome MD (2010, Mar. 25). Untangling the Web — Patients, Doctors, and the Internet. *New England Journal of Medicine* [online]. Retrieved from http://content.nejm.org/cgi/content/full/362/12/1063

68) HIMSS (2002, May). E-Health: Navigating The Internet For Health Information. *Healthcare*

Information and Management Systems Society [online]. Retrieved from http://www.himss.org/content/files/whitepapers/e-health.pdf

69) Risk, Ahmad and Dzenowagis, Joan (2001). Review of Internet Health Information Quality Initiatives. *Journal of Medical Internet Research* [online]. Retrieved from http://www.jmir.org/2001/4/e28/

70) Medline Plus (2010). Evaluating Health Information. *National Library of Medicine* [online]. Retrieved from http://www.nlm.nih.gov/medlineplus/evaluatinghealthinformation.html

71) Medline Plus (2010). Medlineplus Guide to Healthy Web Surfing. *National Library of Medicine* [online]. Retrieved from http://www.nlm.nih.gov/medlineplus/healthywebsurfing.html

72) NCI (2010). Evaluating Health Information on the Internet. *National Cancer Institute* [online]. Retrieved from http://www.cancer.gov/cancertopics/factsheet/Information/internet

73) CSPI (2010). Non-Profit Organizations With Ties to Industry. *Center for Science in the Pubic Interest Integrity in Science Project* [online]. Retrieved from http://www.cspinet.org/integrity/corp_funding.html

74) NSF (2010). About NSF. *The National Sleep Foundation* [online]. Retrieved from http://www.sleepfoundation.org/primary-links/about-nsf

75) MLA (2010). For Health Consumers: "Top Ten" Most Useful Websites. *Medical Library Association* [online]. Retrieved from http://www.mlanet.org/resources/medspeak/topten.html

76) MLA (2010). 2010 CAPHIS Top 100 List Health Websites You Can Trust. *Medical Library Association* [online]. Retrieved from http://caphis.mlanet.org/consumer/top100all.pdf

77) CAPHIS (2010). CAPHIS Top 100: General Health. *Medical Library Association* [online]. Retrieved from http://caphis.mlanet.org/consumer/generalhealth.html

78) MLA (2010). CAPHIS Top 100: Women's Health. *Medical Library Association* [online]. Retrieved from http://caphis.mlanet.org/consumer/womenshealth.html

79) MLA (2010). CAPHIS Top 100: Men's Health. *Medical Library Association* [online]. Retrieved from http://caphis.mlanet.org/consumer/menshealth.html

80) MLA (2010). CAPHIS Top 100: Parenting. *Medical Library Association* [online]. Retrieved from http://caphis.mlanet.org/consumer/parenting.html

81) MLA (2010). CAPHIS Top 100: Senior Health. *Medical Library Association* [online]. Retrieved from http://caphis.mlanet.org/consumer/seniorhealth.html

82) MLA (2010). CAPHIS Top 100: Specific Health. *Medical Library Association* [online]. Retrieved from http://caphis.mlanet.org/consumer/specifichealth.html

83) MLA (2010). CAPHIS Top 100: For Health Professionals. *Medical Library Association* [online]. Retrieved from http://caphis.mlanet.org/consumer/healthprof.html

84) MLA (2010). CAPHIS Top 100: Drug Information. *Medical Library Association* [online]. Retrieved from http://caphis.mlanet.org/consumer/druginfo.html

85) MLA (2010). CAPHIS Top 100: Other Health. *Medical Library Association* [online]. Retrieved from http://caphis.mlanet.org/consumer/otherhealth.html

86) PHR Reviews (2010). Personal Health Record. *Personal Health Record Reviews* [online]. Retrieved from http://www.phrreviews.com/

87) My PHR (2010). What is a PHR? *AHIMA* [online]. Retrieved from http://www.myphr.com/index.php/start_a_phr/what_is_a_phr/

88) AHIMA (2010). Helping Consumers Select PHRs: Questions and Considerations for Navigating an Emerging Market. *AHIMA* [online]. Retrieved from http://library.ahima.org/xpedio/groups/public/documents/ahima/bok1_032260.hcsp?dDocName=bok1_032260

89) Brewster, Anne MD (2009, Oct. 5). Health-Reform Anxiety: One Doctor's Perspective. *Common Health* [online]. Retrieved from http://commonhealth.wbur.org/guest-contributors/2009/10/health-reform-anxiety-one-doctors-perspective/

90) Pho, Kevin (2008). Why Doctors Still Balk at Electronic Medical Records. *USA Today* [online]. Retrieved from http://blogs.usatoday.com/oped/2008/10/why-doctors-sti.html

91) O'Malley AS; Cohen GR and Grossman JM (2010, April). Electronic Medical Records and Communication with Patients and Other Clinicians: Are We Talking Less? *Health System Change* [online]. Retrieved from http://www.hschange.org/CONTENT/1125/

92) Conn, Joseph (2010, Apr. 12). Physician resistance to EHRs weakening: report. *Modern Health Care* [online]. Retrieved from http://www.modernhealthcare.com/article/20100412/NEWS/304129961/1153#

93) Huslin, Anita (2009, Feb. 16). Online Health Data in Remission:
Nascent Industry Ready With Systems If Money and Standards Are Resolved. *The Washington Post* [online]. Retrieved from http://www.washingtonpost.com/wp-dyn/content/article/2009/02/15/AR2009021501284.html

94) My PHR (2010). Common Privacy Myths. *AHIMA* [online]. Retrieved from http://www.myphr.com/index.php/privacy_and_phrs/common_privacy_myths/

95) PHR Reviews (2010). Personal Health Record. *Personal Health Record Reviews* [online]. Retrieved from http://www.phrreviews.com/

96) Google (2010). Frequently Asked Questions. *Google Health* [online]. Retrieved from http://www.google.com/intl/en-US/health/faq.html#phr

97) Resources Shelf Blog (2009, Oct. 5). Your Own Health Info Available Online: Microsoft Releases MyHealthInfo (Beta). *Resources Shelf* [online]. Retrieved from http://www.resourceshelf.com/2009/10/05/microsoft-releases-beta-myhealthinfo/

98) Gearon, Christopher (2005, Mar. 15). A Personal Record: While Feds Delay, Some Digitize Their Own Medical Records. *The Washington Post* [online]. Retrieved from http://www.

washingtonpost.com/ac2/wp-dyn/A35059-2005Mar14?language=printer

99) 911 Medical ID (2010). Maker of Revolutionary USB Portable Personal Health Record Card Introduces New 911 Medical ID Medallion. *911 Medical ID blog* [online]. Retrieved from http://blog.911medicalid.com/2010/01/memitech-releases-new-911-medical-id-medallion/

100) Business Wire (2010, Feb. 16). Office Ally's Focus on Connecting Providers, Patients and Health Plans Continues to Fuel Record-Breaking Growth. *Business Wire* [online]. Retrieved from http://www.businesswire.com/portal/site/home/permalink/?ndmViewId=news_view&newsId=20100216005757&newsLang=en

101) EHNAC (2010). Index. *Electronic Healthcare Network Accreditation Commission* [online]. Retrieved from http://www.ehnac.org/index.html

102) EHNAC (2010). Application Service Provider Accreditation Program for Electronic Health Records (ASPAP-EHR). *Electronic Healthcare Network Accreditation Commission* [online]. Retrieved from http://www.ehnac.org/accreditation-programs/aspap-ehr-accreditation.html

103) EHNAC (2010). Health Information Exchange Accreditation Program (HIEAP). *Electronic Healthcare Network Accreditation Commission* [online]. Retrieved from http://

www.ehnac.org/accreditation-programs/hieap-accreditation.html

104) EHNAC (2010). Healthcare Network Accreditation Program (HNAP). *Electronic Healthcare Network Accreditation Commission* [online]. Retrieved from http://www.ehnac.org/accreditation-programs/hnap-accreditation.html

105) EHNAC (2010). Healthcare Network Accreditation Program (HNAP-70). *Electronic Healthcare Network Accreditation Commission* [online]. Retrieved from http://www.ehnac.org/accreditation-programs/hnap-70-accreditation.html

106) Bentley, Lora (2009, Dec. 3).Privacy Rights Grades Online Health Record Providers on Protections. *IT Business Edge* [online]. Retrieved from http://www.itbusinessedge.com/cm/blogs/bentley/patient-privacy-rights-grades-online-health-record-providers-on-protections/?cs=37862

107) AHIMA (2010). My PHR. *American Health Information Management Association* [online]. Retrieved from http://www.myphr.com/

108) Red Orbit (2008, Feb. 25). CapMed Introduces icePHR Mobile, Allowing Consumers to Access Personal Health Records (PHRs) From Cell Phones. *Redorbit* [online]. Retrieved from http://www.redorbit.com/news/

health/1268077/capmed_introduces_icephr_
mobile_allowing_consumers_to_access_per-
sonal_health/index.html

109) Business Week (2008-2010). Health Trio, LLC. *Business Week* [online]. Retrieved from http://investing.businessweek.com/research/stocks/private/snapshot.asp?privcapId=4773380

110) VMW (2007, Jul. 22). Personal Health Record (PHR) Systems: An Evolving Challenge to EHR Systems. *Virtual Medical Worlds* [online]. Retrieved from http://www.hoise.com/vmw/07/articles/vmw/LV-VM-08-07-26.html

111) Medical News (2007, Jul. 9). ICW America and Memorial Hospital of Rhode Island team up to offer an interoperable personal health record. *The Medical News* [online]. Retrieved from http://www.newsmedical.net/news/2007/07/09/27310.aspx

112) Ficco, Kathy (2006). Mi VIA: Using Technology to Improve Health for Agricultural Workers. *Mobile Health Clinics Network* [online]. Retrieved from http://www.mobilehealthclinic-snetwork.org/sample_abstracts06.html

113) IU News (2009, Feb. 23). Indiana University Health Center launches NoMoreClipboard.com online personal health record. *Indiana University* [online]. Retrieved from http://news-info.iu.edu/news/page/normal/10006.html

114) CAQH (2010) CORE Rules Certification/ Endorsement. *CAQH* [online]. Retrieved from http://www.caqh.org/CORE_certification.php

115) CCHIT (2010). About CCHIT and Learn More About CCHIT's Certification Programs. *Certification Commission for Health Information Technology* [online]. Retrieved from http:// www.cchit.org/

116) Hardy, Kyle (2009, Nov. 18). Practice Fusion launches new PHR. *Healthcare IT News* [online]. Retrieved from http://www.healthcareitnews.com/news/practice-fusion-launches-new-phr

117) Passport MD (2010). Overview of Services. *Passport MD* [online]. Retrieved from http:// www.passportmd.com/services.php

118) Sybert, Laurie (2004, Sept. 3). Doctors' $2.5M launches Vital Vault record depository. *St. Louis Business Journal* [online]. Retrieved from http://www.bizjournals.com/stlouis/stories/2004/09/06/story8.html

119) Moore, John (2007, Oct. 12). Digging Into Microsoft's HealthVault: Part Two (a) – The Platform. *Chilmark Research* [online]. Retrieved from http://chilmarkresearch.com/2007/10/12/digging-into-microsoft%e2%80%99s-healthvault-part-two-a-%e2%80%93-the-platform/

120) Berthold, Jessica (2009). Do Placebos Have a Place in Clinical Practice? *ACP Internist* [online]. Retrieved from http://www.acpinternist.org/archives/2009/04/placebo.htm

121) Miller, Franklin G and Kaptchuk, Ted J (2008). The power of context: reconceptualizing the placebo effect. *Journal of the Royal Society of Medicine* [online]. Retrieved from http://jrsm.rsmjournals.com/cgi/content/full/101/5/222

123) FitzGerald, Sumei and Risholmen, Sondre (2009). Placebo Effect Contextual Healing. *Web Psychologen* [online]. Retrieved from http://www.webpsykologen.no/artikler/psykologi-i-kultur-og-samfunn/placebo-effekten-som-kontekstuell-helbredelse/

124) The Physician's Foundation (2008, November 18). National Survey Finds Numerous Problems Facing Primary Care Doctors, Predicts Escalating Shortage Ahead. *The Physician's Foundation* [online]. Retrieved from http://www.physiciansfoundations.org/PressReleaseDetails.aspx?id=75

125) The Physician's Foundation (2008). The Physician's Perspective: Medical Practice in 2008: Executive Summary. *The Physician's Foundation* [online]. Retrieved from http://www.physiciansfoundations.org/uploadedFiles/News and Publications/Press Releases/Executive Summary for Website.pdf

126) Linzer, Mark and Konrad, Thomas R. (2008, April). Time Pressure Leaves Doctors Dissatisfied. *Generalist Provider Research Initiative* [online]. Retrieved from http://www.rwjf.org/reports/grr/027069.htm

127) Sataline, Suzanne and Wang, Shirley S (2010, Apr. 12). Medical Schools Can't Keep Up. *Wall Street Journal* [online. Retrieved from http://online.wsj.com/article/SB100014240527 02304506904575180331528424238.html

128) LeBlanc, Steve (2009, September 13). Critical need: More primary care doctors for projected surge of 50 million uninsured patients. *ABC News* [online]. Retrieved from http://abcnews.go.com/US/wireStory?id=8562204

129) Kavilanz, Parija B. (2009, September 30). Rx for money woes: Doctors quit medicine. *CNNMoney* [online]. Retrieved from http://money.cnn.com/2009/09/14/news/economy/health_care_doctors_quitting/index.htm

130) Interviewer/writer All Things Considered. (2009). Doctors Say Costs, Not Care, Have Become Focus. Interview with Dr. Greg Darrow and Dr. George Knaysi on *National Public Radio.* June 30, 2009. Retrieved from http://www.npr.org/templates/story/story.php?storyId=10610 0326&ft=1&f=106181580

131) Chen, Pauline W. (2009, October 1). When the Doctor Is Distressed. *New York Times* [online]. Retrieved from http://www.nytimes.com/2009/10/01/health/01chen.html?_r=1

132) Tillet, Richard (2003). The patient within—psychopathology in the helping professions. *The Royal College of Psychiatrists, Advances in Psychiatric Treatment* [online], 9: 272-279. Retrieved from http://apt.rcpsych.org/cgi/content/full/9/4/272

133) Friedenberg, Richard M. (2002, October 16). Patient-Doctor Relationships. *Radiologyrsna.org.* Retrieved from http://radiology.rsna.org/content/226/2/306.full

134) Relman, AS (1994). The impact of market forces on the physician-patient relationship. *Journal of the Royal Society of Medicine* [online] 87:22 Retrieved from, http://www.ncbi.nlm.nih.gov/pmc/articles/PMC1294193/?tool=pubmed

135) Lown, Bernard (2007). The Commodification of Health Care. *Physicians for a National Health Program* [online]. Retrieved from http://www.pnhp.org/publications/the_commodification_of_health_care.php?page=all

136) McKalip, David MD (2009, Jun. 25). An Open Letter to America's Physicians. *Take Back Medicine* [online]. Retrieved from http://www.

takebackmedicine.com/from-david-mckalip-md/

137) Haberkorn, Jennifer (2009, Nov. 17). GOP physicians fear health bill. *The Washington Times* [online]. Retrieved from http://www.washingtontimes.com/news/2009/nov/17/gop-physicians-fear-health-bill/

138) Sullivan, Thomas (2009, Apr. 8). The Pitfalls of Cookbook Medicine. *Policy and Medicine* [online]. Retrieved from http://www.policymed.com/2009/04/the-pitfalls-of-cookbook-medicine.html

139) Groopman, Jerome B and Hartzband, Pamela (2009, Apr. 8). Why 'Quality' Care Is Dangerous. *The Wall Street Journal* [online]. Retrieved from http://online.wsj.com/article/SB123914878625199185.html

140) Court, Jamie and Smith, Francis (2002). **Making a Killing: HMO's and The Threat to Your Health**—Chapter 6: The Battle to Make Health Care Work. *Common Courage Press.* Retrieved from http://www.makingakilling.org/chapter6.html

141) Mayo Clinic (2009). A Perspective on Current Health Reform Issues From Mayo Clinic. *Letter to the Senate/Ted Kaufman* [online]. Retrieved from http://kaufman.senate.gov/press/floor

statements/statement/?id=930aeba3-8128-4226-b99e-db8fb83520a1

142) McCarthy, Douglas, Mueller, Kimberly and Wrenn, Jennifer (2009, Jul. 7). Mayo Clinic: Multidisciplinary Teamwork, Physician-Led Governance, and Patient-Centered Culture Drive World-Class Health Care. *The Commonwealth Fund* [online]. Retrieved from http://www.commonwealthfund.org/Content/Publications/Case-Studies/2009/Aug/Mayo-Clinic-Multidisciplinary-Teamwork-Physician-Led-Governance-and-Patient-Centered-Culture.aspx

143) Mayo Clinic (2010). The Tradition and Heritage of Mayo Clinic. *The Mayo Clinic* [online]. Retrieved from http://www.mayoclinic.org/tradition-heritage/

144) Waggoner, Judy (2000, Apr. 25). Doctors outside insurance. *Marketplace* [online]. Retrieved from http://www.allbusiness.com/specialty-businesses/1123000-1.html

145) Flanagan, Lyndia (1998). Nurse Practitioners: Growing Competition for Family Physicians? *American Academy of Family Physicians* [online]. Retrieved from http://www.aafp.org/fpm/981000fm/nurse.html

146) Horrocks, Sue; Anderson, Elizabeth; and Salisbury, Chris (2002, Apr. 6). Systematic

review of whether nurse practitioners working in primary care can provide equivalent care to doctors. *British Medical Journal* [online]. Retrieved from http://www.bmj.com/cgi/content/abstract/bmj;324/7341/819

147) Bryre G; Richardson M; Brundson J; Patel A (2001, Dec. 24). Patient satisfaction with emergency nurse practitioners in A & E . *Journal of Clinical Nursing* [online]. Retrieved from http://www3.interscience.wiley.com/journal/119188466/abstract

148) Hooker, Roderick A (2006, Jul. 3). Physician assistants and nurse practitioners: the United States experience. *Medical Journal of Australia* [online]. Retrieved from https://www.mja.com.au/public/issues/185_01_030706/hoo10101_fm.pdf

149) Rough, Ginger (2009, Feb. 21). For many, a nurse practitioner is the doctor. *The Arizona Republic* [online]. Retrieved from http://www.azcentral.com/news/articles/2009/02/21/20090221nursepractitioners0220.html

150) Lofton, Lynn (2008, Jun. 23). Nurse practitioners helping fill primary care void in state. *The Mississippi Business Journal* [online]. Retrieved from http://www.allbusiness.com/health-care/health-care-professionals-nurses-nursing/11466281-1.html

151) Rodriguez, Maggies (2009, Jul 6). Retail Clinic Route Best Low-Cost Care? *CBS News* [online]. Retrieved from http://www.cbsnews. com/stories/2009/07/06/earlyshow/health/ main5136763.shtml

152) Health Behavior News Service (2008, August). Retail Clinics: What's in Store for Health Care. *Center for Advancing Health: The Prepared Patient* [online]. Retrieved from http://www.cfah.org/hbns/preparedpatient/ Prepared-Patient-Vol1-Issue10.cfm

153) Health Behavior News Service (2007, October). Chronic Conditions: When Do You Call the Doctor? *Center for Advancing Health: The Prepared Patient* [online]. Retrieved from http://www.cfah.org/hbns/preparedpatient/ Prepared-Patient-Vol1-Issue2.cfm

154) Kalogredis, Vasilios J. JD (2004, February). Should you consider concierge medicine? *Physician News* [online]. Retrieved from http:// www.physiciansnews.com/business/204.kalo- gredis.html

155) Wahlgren, Eric (2010, Feb. 10). Concierge Medicine: Patients Pay Up for a Doctor's Undivided Attention. *Daily Finance* [online]. Retrieved from http://www.dailyfinance.com/ story/concierge-medicine-patients-pay-up-for- a-doctors-undivided-att/19349963/

156) History Link Staff (2005, Aug. 9). Health care reformer Dr. Michael Shadid speaks to future founders of Group Health Cooperative in Seattle on August 14, 1945. *History Link* [online]. Retrieved from http://www.historylink. org/index.cfm?DisplayPage=output.cfm&file id=7411

157) Leonhardt, David (2009, Jul. 25). Forget Who Pays Medical Bills, It's Who Sets the Cost. *The New York Times* [online]. Retrieved from http://www.nytimes.com/2009/07/26/ weekinreview/26leonhardt.html

158) Hess, Corrinne (2010, Apr. 9). Firms consider concierge care to save costs. *The Business Journal of Milwaukee* [online]. Retrieved from http://milwaukee.bizjournals. com/milwaukee/stories/2010/04/12/story2. html?b=1271044800%5E3169281

159) Parker-Pope, Tara (2010, Apr. 8). Paperwork vs. Patients. *The New York Times* [online]. Retrieved from http://well.blogs.nytimes. com/2010/04/08/paperwork-vs-patients/

160) Chen, Pauline W. MD (2010, Apr. 8). Doctors and Patients, Lost in Paperwork. *The New York Times* [online]. Retrieved from http://www. nytimes.com/2010/04/08/health/08chen.html

161) PNHP (2010). Our Mission: Single-Payer National Health Insurance. *Physicians for a*

National Health Program [online]. Retrieved from http://www.pnhp.org/

162) Keith, Tamara (2009, Jan. 22). The controversy of concierge medicine. *American Public Media: Marketplace* [online]. Retrieved from http://marketplace.publicradio.org/display/web/2009/01/22/concierge_medicine/

163) Sonn, Bill (2004, February). Concierge Medicine: Physicians Weigh Financial, Ethical Issues. *Physician's Practice* [online]. Retrieved from http://www.physicianspractice.com/index/fuseaction/articles.details/articleID/483.htm

164) Lindsay, Drew (2010, Feb. 1). Concierge Medicine. *The Washingtonian* [online]. Retrieved from http://www.washingtonian.com/articles/health/14750.html

165) Rangel MD (2010, Mar. 12). Top 9 Criticisms of Concierge Medicine. *RangelMD* [online]. Retrieved from http://rangelmd.com/2010/03/top-7-criticisms-of-concierge-medicine/

166) DHCS (2008). The Medical Home: Disruptive Innovation for a New Primary Care Model. *Deloitte Center for Health Solutions* [online]. Retrieved from http://www.dhcs.ca.gov/provgovpart/Documents/Deloitte%20-%20Financial%20Model%20for%20Medical%20Home.pdf

167) CDC (2009). Chronic Diseases: The Power to Prevent, The Call to Control: At a Glance 2009. *Centers for Disease Control and Prevention* [online]. Retrieved from http://www. cdc.gov/chronicdisease/resources/publications/ AAG/chronic.htm

168) AAFP, AAP, ACP, AOA (2007, March). Joint Principles of the Patient-Centered Medical Home. *American College of Physicians* [online]. Retrieved from http://www.acponline.org/running practice/pcmh/demonstrations/joint-princ 05 17.pdf

169) ACP (2010). What is the Patient-Centered Medical Home? *The American College of Physicians* [online]. Retrieved from http://www. acponline.org/running practice/pcmh/understanding/what.htm

170) Davis, Henry L. (2010, Feb. 6). The 'medical home' experiment: Team concept seeks to improve basic care. *Buffalo News* [online]. Retrieved from http://www.buffalonews. com/2010/02/05/947496/the-medical-home-experiment.html

171) PCPCC (2010). Evaluation/Evidence of PCMH *Patient-Centered Primary Care Collaborative* [online]. Retrieved from http://www. pcpcc.net/evaluation-evidence

172) UPI (2010, Mar. 19). Pediatric medical home effective. *United Press International* [online]. Retrieved from http://www.upi.com/ Health_News/2010/03/19/Pediatric-medical-home-effective/UPI-21311269053501/

173) NCCAM (2009, April). Are You Considering CAM? *National Center for Complementary and Alternative Medicine* [online]. Retrieved from http://nccam.nih.gov/health/decisions/consideringcam.htm

174) WHO (2008, December). Traditional medicine. *World Health Organization* [online]. Retrieved from http://www.who.int/mediacentre/factsheets/fs134/en/

175) NCCAM (2009, Oct. 26). Ayurveda: An Introduction. *National Center for Complementary and Alternative Medicine* [online]. Retrieved from http://nccam.nih.gov/health/ayurveda/introduction.htm

176) NCCAM (2009, Nov. 11). Traditional Chinese Medicine: An Introduction. *National Center for Complementary and Alternative Medicine* [online]. Retrieved from http://nccam.nih.gov/health/whatiscam/chinesemed.htm

177) NCCAM (2009, Oct. 13). Homeopathy: An Introduction. *National Center for Complementary and Alternative Medicine* [online].

Retrieved from http://nccam.nih.gov/health/homeopathy/

178) NCCAM (2007, April). An Introduction to Naturopathy. *National Center for Complementary and Alternative Medicine* [online]. Retrieved from http://nccam.nih.gov/health/naturopathy/

179) Ehrlich, Steven D. NMD (2009, Sept. 29). Naturopathy. *University of Maryland Medical Center* [online]. Retrieved from http://www.umm.edu/altmed/articles/naturopathy-000356.htm

180) ACS (2008, Nov. 1) Naturopathic Medicine. *American Cancer Society* [online]. Retrieved from http://www.cancer.org/docroot/ETO/content/ETO_5_3X_Naturopathic_Medicine.asp

181) Erlich, Steven D. NMD (2009, Sept. 27). Herbal Medicine. *University of Maryland Medical Center* [online]. Retrieved from http://www.umm.edu/altmed/articles/herbal-medicine-000351.htm

182) Vickers, Andrew and Zollman, Catherine (1999, Oct. 16). Clinical Review: ABC of Complementary Medicine: Herbal Medicine. *British Medical Journal* [online]. Retrieved from http://www.bmj.com/cgi/content/full/319/7216/1050

183) ODS (2009, Jul. 9). Botanical Dietary Supplements: Background Information. *Office of*

Dietary Supplements [online]. Retrieved from http://ods.od.nih.gov/factsheets/Botanical-Background.asp

184) Mayo Clinic (2009, Jul. 9). Herbal supplements: What to know before you buy. *Mayo Clinic* [online]. Retrieved from http://www.mayoclinic.com/health/herbalsupplements/SA00044/METHOD=print

185) Preidt, Robert (2010, Apr. 8). Insight on Herbals Eludes Doctors, Patients Alike. *Medline Plus* [online]. Retrieved from http://www.nlm.nih.gov/medlineplus/news/fullstory_97377.html

186) Walter, Suzan (2010). **The Illustrated Encyclopedia of Body-Mind Disciplines** excerpt: Holistic Health. *American Holistic Health Association* [online]. Retrieved from http://ahha.org/articles.asp?Id=85

187) Walter, Suzan (2010). Holistic is an Adjective...Not a Noun. *American Holistic Health Association* [online]. Retrieved from http://ahha.org/articles.asp?Id=86

188) Ivker, Robert S. DO (2010). Comparing Holistic and Conventional Medicine. *American Holistic Health Association* [online]. Retrieved from http://ahha.org/articles.asp?Id=38

189) Miller, Robert 2010, Mar. 29). Treating pain, holistically. *News Times* [online]. Retrieved from http://www.newstimes.com/news/article/Treating-pain-holistically-427388.php

190) Duke Integrative Medicine (2009). About Us: What is Integrative Medicine? *Duke University* [online]. Retrieved from http://www.dukeintegrativemedicine.org/index.php/2009011913/about-us/what-is-integrative-medicine.html

191) Boniol, Leti (2010, Apr. 10). Are You Ready for Integrative Medicine? *Phillipine Daily Inquirer* [online]. Retrieved from http://showbizandstyle.inquirer.net/sim/sim/view/20100410-263419/Are-You-Ready-for-Integrative-Medicine

192) Frontline Interview (2003, Nov. 4). Pros and Cons of Integrative Medicine. *PBS* [online]. Retrieved from http://www.pbs.org/wgbh/pages/frontline/shows/altmed/clash/integrated.html

193) All Business (2010). The Facts about PPO, HMO, FFS, and POS Plans. *All Business* [online]. Retrieved from http://www.allbusiness.com/human-resources/benefits-insurance-health-types/770-1.html

194) 194)AHA (2010). Managed Health Care Plans. *American Heart Association* [online]. Retrieved from http://www.americanheart.org/presenter.jhtml?identifier=4663

195) Schwab Money Wise (2010). Group Health Insurance: HMOs, PPOs and POSs: Understanding your options and choosing the right plan. *Charles Schwab* [online]. Retrieved from http://www.schwabmoneywise.com/basics/insurance/group-health-insurance.php

196) Schwab Money Wise (2010). Individual Health Insurance: Going it alone. *Charles Schwab* [online]. Retrieved from http://www.schwabmoneywise.com/basics/insurance/individual-health-insurance.php

197) Science Daily (2009, Jun. 5). Over 60 Percent Of All US Bankruptcies Attributable To Medical Problems. *Elsevier Health Sciences* [online]. Retrieved from http://www.sciencedaily.com/releases/2009/06/090604095123.htm

198) WHO (2000, June). World Health Organization Assesses the World's Health Systems. *World Health Organization* [online]. Retrieved from http://www.photius.com/rankings/who world health ranks.html

199) Mahon, Mary (April 4, 2006). New Cross-National Comparisons of Health Systems: US Ranks Lowest in Patient Surveys, Has Greatest Inequity for Lower-Income Patients. *The Commonwealth Fund* [online]. Retrieved from http://www.commonwealthfund.org/Content/News/News-Releases/2006/Apr/New-Cross-National-

Comparisons-of-Health-Systems–U-S–Ranks-Lowest-in-Patient-Surveys–Has-Greatest.aspx

200) Dunham, Will (January 8, 2008): "U.S. Ranks 19th in Preventable Deaths" *Reuters* [online]. Retrieved from http://www.reuters.com/article/idUSN0765165020080108

201) RWJF (2009, Jun. 8). New Poll Finds Disease Prevention is Top Priority for Americans in Health Reform. *Robert Wood Johnson Foundation* [online]. Retrieved from http://www.rwjf.org/publichealth/product.jsp?id=44536

202) "Chronic Diseases and Health Promotion;" (2010): *World Health Organization* [online]. Retrieved from http://www.who.int/chp/en/index.html

203) "Diet and Physical Activity: a public health priority;" (2010): *World Health Organization* [online]. Retrieved from http://www.who.int/dietphysicalactivity/en/index.html

204) Reid, T.R. (August 23, 2009): "5 Myths About Health Care Around the World;"*Washington Post* [online]. Retrieved from http://www.washingtonpost.com/wp-dyn/content/article/2009/08/21/AR2009082101778_pf.html

205) England, Mary Jane (2007, December 3): "Diagnosing U.S. Health Care" *American Magazine* [online]. Retrieved from http://www.amer-

icamagazine.org/content/article.cfm?article id=10452&comments=1

206) Bass, Sarah Bauerle et al. (2006, March). Relationship of Internet Health Information Use With Patient Behavior and Self-Efficacy: Experiences of Newly Diagnosed Cancer Patients Who Contact the National Cancer Institute's Cancer Information Service. *Journal of Health Communications* [online]. Retrieved from http://www.informaworld.com/smpp/content~db=all~content=a742065861

207) Fox, Susannah and Jones, Syndey (2009, Jun. 11). The Social Life of Health Information. *Pew Internet* [online]. Retrieved from http://www.pewinternet.org/Reports/2009/8-The-Social-Life-of-Health-Information.aspx

208) Miller, Claire Cain (2010, Mar. 24). Social Networks a Lifeline for the Chronically Ill. *The New York Times* [online]. Retrieved from http://www.nytimes.com/2010/03/25/technology/25disable.html

209) Fox, Susannah (2009, Oct. 6). The Patient is In. *Pew Internet Project* [online]. Retrieved from http://www.pewinternet.org/Presentations/2009/30–The-Patient-is-In.aspx